S0-BPY-928

LANGLEY PORTER
PSYCHIATRIC INSTITUTE
LIBRARY

PRIMARY PREVENTION IN PSYCHIATRY:

STATE OF THE ART

LANGLEY PORTER
PSYCHIATRIC INSTITUTE
LIBRARY

PRIMARY PREVENTION IN PSYCHIATRY:

STATE OF THE ART

Edited by

JAMES T. BARTER, M.D.

and

SUSAN W. TALBOTT, R.N., M.A., M.B.A.

RA 790
P7756
1986

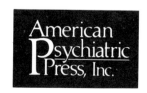
American Psychiatric Press, Inc.

1400 K Street, N.W.
Washington, DC 20005

Books published by the American Psychiatric Press, Inc., represent the views and opinions of the individual authors and do not necessarily reflect the policies and opinions of the Press or the American Psychiatric Association.

Copyright © 1986 American Psychiatric Press, Inc.

ALL RIGHTS RESERVED

Manufactured in the United States of America

Library of Congress Cataloging-in-Publication Data

Primary prevention in psychiatry.

　　Based on a symposium held at the 1985 American Psychiatric Association Annual Meeting in Dallas, Tex.
　　Includes bibliographies.
　　1. Mental illness--Prevention--Congresses. 2. Mental health services--United States--Congresses. 3. Medicine, Preventive--United States--Congresses. I. Barter, James T. II. Talbott, Susan W., 1939-　　. III. American Psychiatric Association. Meeting (138th : 1985 : Dallas, Tex.) [DNLM: 1. Community Mental Health Services--United States--congresses. 2. Mental Disorders--prevention & control--congresses. 3. Primary Prevention--congresses. WM 105 P952 1985]

RA790.P7756　1986　　616.89'05　　86-14134
ISBN 0-88048-130-7 (soft)

Contents

Contributors

Regina Armas, Ph.D.
Research Associate, University of California, San Francisco

Joan R. Asarnow, Ph.D.
Assistant Professor in Residence, Department of Psychiatry and Biobehavioral Sciences, University of California, Los Angeles

Bernard L. Bloom, Ph.D.
Professor of Psychology, University of Colorado, Boulder

Rosalynn Carter
Plains, Georgia

Florentius Chan, Ph.D.
Community Psychologist, Coastal Asian/Pacific Mental Health Services, Department of Mental Health, County of Los Angeles, California

Leon Eisenberg, M.D.
Professor and Chairman, Department of Social Medicine and Health Policy, Harvard Medical School, Boston, Massachusetts

Richard Frances, M.D.
Associate Professor of Clinical Psychiatry, New York Hospital--Cornell Medical Center, Westchester Division, White Plains, New York

John E. Franklin, M.D.
Instructor in Psychiatry, New York Hospital--Cornell Medical Center, Westchester Division, White Plains, New York

Michael J. Goldstein, Ph.D.
Professor of Psychology, University of California, Los Angeles

Donald I. Macdonald, M.D.
Administrator, Alcohol, Drug Abuse, and Mental Health Administration, National Institute of Mental Health, Rockville, Maryland

Ricardo F. Munoz, Ph.D.
Associate Professor of Psychology, University of California,
San Francisco

Joaquim Puig-Antich, M.D.
Chief, Child and Adolescent Psychiatry, Western Psychiatric
Institute and Clinic, University of Pittsburgh, Pennsylvania

Steven S. Sharfstein, M.D.
Deputy Medical Director, American Psychiatric Association,
Washington, DC

Kenneth Tardiff, M.D., M.P.H.
Associate Professor of Psychiatry and of Public Health,
Cornell University Medical College, New York

Foreword

My interest in the public policy aspects of mental health care dates back to 1970 when my husband, Jimmy Carter, became governor of Georgia. One of the first things he did was set up a special study commission to advise him on how to improve Georgia's mental health system. He appointed me a member of the commission, and this gave me an opportunity to learn firsthand about the organization and delivery of mental health services.

In 1977, when Jimmy became President, I selected mental health as my major area of interest, with hopes of improving the care of the mentally ill throughout the country. We began with the creation of the President's Commission on Mental Health. Our 1978 Report to the President represented the first comprehensive review of the nation's mental health system and its needs since the 1961 Report of the Joint Commission on Mental Illness and Health presented to President John F. Kennedy.

In our year-long study, it became clear that the needs of the mentally ill far exceeded the resources available to meet them and that new approaches would be necessary if society were to have any hope of meeting those needs in the future.

This kind of reasoning led us to stress the need to develop means for preventing mental and emotional disorders. In 1978, we called for increased commitment to and investment in preventive strategies. That call is just as urgent today.

This monograph represents a broad overview of the state of the art of prevention of mental disorders. It focuses on what is known, what works, and what can be done. I hope that it will stimulate thoughtful consideration of the issues involved in the prevention of mental illnesses and lend inspiration for continued work in this vital aspect of mental health care.

Rosalynn Carter

Introduction

This monograph originated in a symposium held at the 1985 annual meeting of the American Psychiatric Association. The contributors wanted to concentrate on the issue of primary prevention in psychiatry as a counterbalance to the clinical, research, and scientific papers that dealt mainly with the treatment of mental illness or its biochemical mysteries. In spite of the gloomy and negativistic pronouncements of the Lamb and Zusman paper of 1979 (1), we felt there was value in presenting the best work currently being done in the area of primary prevention, emphasizing the practical aspects of "What do we know?"; "What works?"; and "What more can be done?" Participating in this symposium were experts on various aspects of prevention who provided a wide range of subject matter. Because of their excellence, these presentations deserve a wider audience.

Prevention of mental disorders is not an esoteric topic. A wide variety of mental disorders exist that can be prevented, including those induced by poisons, infections, nutritional deficiencies, endocrine imbalances, and injuries to the central nervous system as well as those with a genetic etiology. All of these etiologies continue to be seen in clinical practice and when recognized and managed successfully can prevent mental illness. An example of this kind of primary prevention is to eliminate lead in the environment of children to prevent the development of the mental symptoms associated with plumbism. This is referred to as a specific disease paradigm in which there is a known etiology whose effect can be ameliorated by the proper intervention. Unfortunately, for the major mental disorders there is no known specific etiology that can be eliminated or dealt with to prevent the disorder. Recognition of this has led to the development of a general approach to prevention that is based on the idea of reducing mental disorders through effective control of stress. In an overview of primary prevention of mental disorders in Chapter 1, Dr. Bernard Bloom discusses this shift in approach and the implications of various prevention strategies built on early intervention to decrease the impact of stressful life events or to increase coping abilities through social competence building or changing the level of social support available to the individual. Although this strategy has been successful, there are formidable barriers, as Dr. Bloom points out, to widespread adoption of these techniques, the most significant of which is failure to allocate sufficient resources to prevention efforts. Perhaps we are the victims of a reimbursement system that is geared toward payment for treating rather than preventing illness.

In Chapter 2, Drs. Ricardo Munoz, Florentius Chan, and Regina Armas present an overview of primary prevention of mental disorders from a cross-cultural perspective. Included in their extensive scope is not only the theoretical issues for prevention across cultures but also discussion of the prevention intervention strategies currently used with the major ethnic groups in this country. A particularly important point is raised in their discussion of Dr. Hayes-Bautista's (2) analysis of the changing shape of the population pyramid for ethnic groups in California. If this interpretation is correct, by the early years of the next century a major role reversal will have occurred, with a largely elderly white minority population being supported by ethnic majorities. The suggestion is made that attention to improvement in race relations now could be a force for prevention of social disability among the elderly then. Finally, recommendations are offered for those interested in working in the primary prevention field that, if followed, would result in improved quality in both research and published results.

An obvious time for primary prevention intervention is during childhood; in Chapter 3 Dr. Leon Eisenberg reviews primary prevention of mental disorders in this context. Prevention of mental disorders is contended to be worthwhile more because it improves health than because it can be cost effective. In fact, Dr. Eisenberg points out, in many instances an increase, not a decrease, in social and financial costs results from prevention interventions. A mistake made by community mental health programs has been to sell alternative community care and treatment as more cost effective, a tenet that could not be proved and is probably wrong because quality care in any setting is more expensive than poor care.

Likewise, prevention should not be oversold as more cost effective or as a panacea. Preventing brain damage and enhancing psychosocial development offer strategies for promoting health in a timely fashion for children, and "better beginnings improve the odds for happier endings."

The growth in our understanding of affective disorders has been substantial in recent years. Even though we are not in a position to specify discrete prevention strategies in this area, there is enough data to point out some approaches. These are comprehensively discussed by Dr. Joaquim Puig-Antich in Chapter 4 on the prevention of depression in children and adolescents. Since episodes of affective disorder predict future episodes, there is an obvious logic to ameliorating or eliminating early-onset dysphoric or affective disorders. Early identification, early intervention, and treatment are obvious approaches, but reducing the use of alcohol and drugs of abuse in familial aggregations that have high density for affective disorders can also be effective.

Probably there is more pessimism about the possibility of effective prevention of schizophrenia than for prevention of any other disorder. Drs. Michael Goldstein and Joan Asarnow comprehensively review the major literature on prevention of schizophrenia by life stage in Chapter 5. They organize a lot of information and make it more comprehensible. One of the more promising approaches to primary prevention, they believe, is to identify individuals at high risk for schizophrenia or schizophrenia-spectrum disorders in the hope of being able to alter the life course of these individuals. Such persons can be identified at virtually every stage of development and the interventions then tailored to that stage. Of interest are the family intervention approaches, which seek to identify high-risk family units using measures of affective style, communication deviance, and expressed emotion. The negative response that these theoretical concepts have evoked in the families of schizophrenics has the potential of hindering the progress of prevention programs based on them.

Efforts to prevent alcohol and other substance abuse have received a great deal of coverage in the media as well as in scientific literature. The disability caused by these substances is largely self induced and is supported by social and cultural norms. The economic consequences of alcohol and substance abuse are enormous and complicated. In Chapter 6 Drs. Richard Frances and John Franklin suggest that a biopsychosocial model of the illness is crucial to the development of prevention strategies. The search for biological markers and social factors can lead to the identification of high-risk populations for whom strategic interventions could be directed. Their overview covers the development of techniques for

identifying high-risk populations, educating the public, and limiting the availability and thus the use of substances. Ultimately, a
significant change in social policy will be needed if prevention of
substance abuse is to be successful.

The loss of lives through homicide and homicide's impact on a
wide segment of the population are characterized by Dr. Kenneth
Tardiff as a major public health problem. His discussion of prevention of homicide identifies what we know about the antecedents of murder and how to prevent it based on that knowledge.
Certainly there are few clear-cut answers (discrete biological
causes are unknown), and some of the data are unreliable and
more a matter of belief system than proven scientific fact. For example, directly contradictory results have been found from studies
on the deterrence effect of execution on preventing homicides.
Some ideas are provocative, such as the use of long-term incarceration to decrease the incidence of homicide and violence. However, the concern over violence dictates that we pay more than lip
service to efforts at prevention, a responsibility that Dr. Tardiff
rightfully contends is "within our area of expertise as mental
health professionals . . . and within our responsibilities as
citizens."

Discussions by Drs. Donald Macdonald and Steven Sharfstein in
Chapters 8 and 9, respectively, increase the dimension of this
work. Dr. Macdonald's discussion of the various ways in which the
Alcohol, Drug Abuse, and Mental Health Administration
(ADAMHA) of the U.S. Department of Health and Human Services has supported preventive efforts across a broad range of
mental health problems confirms the wisdom of establishing a
permanent Associate Administrator for Prevention within
ADAMHA. Dr. Sharfstein's personal reflections on his initial
skepticism about prevention will strike a responsive note for many
readers and serve to remind us that sometimes increased knowledge and a shift in perspective can be enlightening.

Finally, we are indebted to Mrs. Rosalynn Carter for her continued interest in mental health, especially in the area of prevention. To quote Drs. Munoz, Chan, and Armas, regarding primary prevention of mental health disorders, "in the long run,
those who say it can't be done will be silenced by someone doing
it."

James T. Barter, M.D.
Susan W. Talbott, R.N., M.A., M.B.A.

REFERENCES

1. Lamb HR, Zusman J: Primary prevention in perspective. Am J Psychiatry 136:12-17, 1979
2. Hayes-Bautista D: Raza demographics and social policy, in Issues in Latino Health. Symposium conducted at the meeting of the Bay Area Latino Health Sciences Faculty Network, Berkeley, California, March 1983

1

Primary Prevention: An Overview

Bernard L. Bloom, Ph.D.

1

Primary Prevention: An Overview

In the past two years, I have found my thinking shifting from its roots in clinical psychology and community mental health to the larger field of community mental health. This shift is particularly true regarding primary prevention, as it has become obvious to me that almost everything we know about the prevention of mental disorders applies equally to the prevention of physical disorders. Interest in primary prevention is sweeping the entire health service delivery system, and mental health professionals, in my judgment, have important contributions to make to the prevention of all illness, physical as well as mental.

In this chapter, an overview of primary prevention from a public health view is presented and five issues are discussed. These are 1) the growing convergence of the paradigms that govern the thinking of general health professionals and mental health professionals, 2) the growing awareness of the inter-dependence of physical and mental health, 3) the concept of the generic illness that is emerging from contemporary research, 4) the rationale of nonspecific preventive interventions in the fields of both physical and mental health, and 5) the ramifications of the growing understanding of the role of self-destructive life-styles in the development of illness. At the conclusion of the chapter, the specific role of primary prevention in the field of mental health field is examined.

THE PUBLIC HEALTH VIEW OF PREVENTION

In the control of any disorder, emotional or physical, two types of interventions exist. The goal of the first type is to reduce the number of persons who are suffering from the disorder, that is, the prevalence of the disorder. The goal of the second type of intervention is to reduce the severity, discomfort, or disability associated with the disorder.

Programs designed to reduce severity, discomfort, or disability are formally known as *tertiary prevention* but are better known as *rehabilitation*. For lifelong disorders, rehabilitation programs generally have little effect on prevalence. Indeed, a well-run rehabilitation program may actually increase the prevalence of these disorders by increasing life expectancy. Unfortunately, at our current level of knowledge, many emotional disorders appear to be lifelong or nearly lifelong and thus cannot be significantly reduced in prevalence through rehabilitation programs.

Because the prevalence of any disorder is a function of its duration and the rate at which new cases are produced, two approaches to reducing the prevalence of a disorder are commonly identified. The first seeks to reduce prevalence by reducing duration, usually through development of some early case-finding combined with prompt application of effective treatment. This approach is termed *secondary prevention*. Secondary prevention efforts are preventive only in that systematic early case-finding brings with it the possibility of reducing the duration of a disorder.

Should a technique for the early identification of a disorder be developed without concomitant development of more effective treatment procedures, as was the case of improved early identification of diabetes, a paradoxical increase in the prevalence of that disorder would occur (1). A similar increase in the prevalence of Down's syndrome has occurred as a consequence of the development of antibiotics, which have significantly reduced the death rate from secondary causes among persons with this syndrome. Gruenberg (2) described medical advances of this sort as "failures of success."

The alternative approach to prevalence reduction is to reduce the rate at which new cases of a disorder develop. Reduction of prevalence via reduction of incidence is formally termed *primary prevention*. The concept of primary prevention most closely matches the lay use of the term *prevention*. Effective primary prevention programs prevent disorders from occurring in the first place or reduce the likelihood that a disorder will occur in a particular population (3, 4).

CONVERGENCE OF HEALTH AND ILLNESS PARADIGMS

Until perhaps 20 years ago, the prevailing models that guided the work of health care providers were essentially disease specific.

Diseases were thought to differ from each other in terms of causative factors and treatment responsivity, so that for each unique disease a unique means for its prevention and a unique strategy for its treatment were sought. For physical illnesses, the prevailing disease-specific models were biomedical; in the case of mental illnesses, the prevailing disease-specific models were psychodynamic.

Psychodynamic theory was once the great rudder that stabilized and guided our beliefs and actions as students and practitioners. However, it has been eclipsed in the past two decades by the extraordinary rise of biological psychiatry. The current emphasis on biological research is in part a result of increasing awareness of the limited effectiveness of psychotherapy. Many practitioners now look to success in the laboratory rather than success in the consulting office as the best hope for helping the mentally ill.

While psychiatry is being "biologized," general medicine is being "psychologized"--perhaps for the same reason. Just as the psychodynamic approach is perceived as having failed to live up to the hopes of its advocates in the mental health field, the biomedical approach is now perceived as failing to live up to expectations in general medicine.

The research of the past two decades has made a compelling case that there is a biology of health, a psychology of health, and a sociology of health (5-9). Whether in regard to treatment or in regard to prevention, the natural interactions of these three domains must be studied. There is a dramatic trend toward an ecumenical view of health and illness--this view has opened new vistas for each of the core mental health disciplines. Considering that current changes in the organization of medical care may result in mental health and general health services' becoming more integrated, the convergence of physical illness and mental illness paradigms could not have come at a better time.

INTERDEPENDENCE OF
PHYSICAL AND MENTAL HEALTH

The growing convergence of thought regarding physical and mental health is supported by overwhelming evidence that mind and body are linked. As far as vulnerability is concerned, there is clear evidence that mentally ill persons have more physical illness than do persons who are thriving psychologically and that people who are physically ill have a higher risk of developing psychiatric disorders than do those who are physically healthy. Also, regarding remediation, there is evidence that attention to physical well-being increases psychological well-being and vice versa (10-15).

Preventive mental health services in the physical health context, through such programs as psychiatric liaison, are remarkably cost effective--an important consideration in this era of cost containment. The high cost of medical care now justifies virtually any responsible effort at prevention.

THE EMERGENCE OF THE GENERIC ILLNESS

Although the majority of research being conducted to obtain more effective prevention strategies continues to be disease specific, increasing evidence suggests that there is a very strong generic component to illness (16). An example of this generic phenomenon can be found in research regarding stressful life events and social support networks. When persons who are ill are compared with persons who are well, the ill group is generally found to have experienced significantly more recent stress and to have significantly weaker sources of social support than the well group. In contrast, when persons who have a particular illness (almost regardless of whether it's physical or mental) are compared with persons who have another type of illness (again, almost regardless of whether physical or mental), differences are rarely found in prior stress or in the strength of social support networks (17-19).

Thus the evidence suggests that there are no stress-specific disorders. Stress is a factor in the precipitation of a number of illnesses, and a strong social support network reduces the risk of contracting an extraordinary variety of illnesses.

NONSPECIFIC PREVENTIVE INTERVENTIONS

Close examination of contemporary general health preventive intervention programs reveals an important shared characteristic: They focus primarily on strategies that are not disease specific. For example, careful attention to nutritional practice; increased physical activity for persons with relatively sedentary jobs; and reductions in smoking, alcohol consumption, and other drug consumption are emphasized. Efforts to reduce stress are supported by recent research studies in which unmanageable stress has been found to be associated with excess risk of individuals' developing a variety of disorders (20-28).

Other nonspecific mental health components should be introduced into preventive intervention programs. These include building a psychological sense of community (29); increasing self-efficacy (30, 31); and enhancing interpersonal problem-solving skills by using such methods as social competency building, mental health education, and community organizations (32, 33). What is particularly striking about such nonspecific preventive interventions is that they usually result in improved physical health, as well as improved mental health (reviewed in 21).

Many of these nonspecific interventions are educational in nature. This is entirely appropriate. After all, the etymology of the word *doctor* includes the latin word *docere* meaning "to teach." In my judgment, mental health professionals should work to become better teachers and should help those in primary care medicine do the same.

LIFE-STYLE COMPONENTS OF ILL HEALTH

The convergence of thought regarding physical and mental disorders is also related to the role of life-style in the predisposition, precipitation, and perpetuation of illness (34). Of the 10 leading causes of death in the United States, 7 are in large part behaviorally determined (35). Modifying life-style implies modifying attitudes and behavior. Changing attitudes and behavior requires a special set of competencies--competencies that are the domain of the mental health professions and the social sciences.

A recent bibliography of research studies dealing with smoking cessation programs (36) listed approximately 35 papers from around the world in which an extraordinary cost-effective strategy is described and urged. This strategy is for physicians to suggest to their patients that they should stop smoking. Research suggests that if all physicians would take a moment to urge their smoking patients to stop smoking, their aggregate efforts would produce more ex-smokers than do all of the intensive smoking cessation clinics combined (37). The interesting question, again one that social scientists may be especially competent to explore, is, Why do so few physicians make that suggestion?

CONCLUSIONS

The history of medicine is a history of triumphs of disease prevention. For example, smallpox, typhus, cholera, typhoid fever, plaque, malaria, diphtheria, tuberculosis, and tetanus can all be prevented; in addition, measles, polio, and many of the sexually transmitted diseases can be prevented. Among the diseases associated with nutritional deficiencies, many are preventable: scurvy, beriberi, pellagra, rickets, kwashiorkor, and endemic goiter.

Most of these diseases were conquered in a simpler time. The sharp drop in their incidence has led to the development of a far more complex group of chronic conditions, including many emotional disorders. Even so, the successful eradication of these diseases motivates our search for strategies to prevent or ameliorate specific psychiatric diseases.

If we are wise, we will accord equal status to primary prevention programs that are patterned after general health promotion paradigms (38). Health promotion programs are those activities that have a generally salutary but unspecifiable effect on health.

In my judgment, the most effective health promotion programs are to be derived from stressful life event theory. This theory suggests that reducing counterproductive stresses and helping people cope more successfully with stress when it is unavoidable results in generally healthier people who are less vulnerable to illness (21).

My own research experiences and my analysis of the prevention literature leave me with absolutely no doubt that preventive intervention programs derived from stressful life event theory are effective. The work of our group at the University of Colorado in implementing and evaluating a preventive intervention program for persons who are undergoing marital disruption has had such favorable long-term results that it stands as a prototype of what can be accomplished in working with persons undergoing stressful life events (39). In addition, Felner and his colleagues (40) studied the stress of developmental transitions within the school system, Lynch (41) studied the stresses associated with coronary artery disease, and Melamed and Bush (42) studied stresses in children that are precipitated by medical procedures. We have hardly begun to explore the full possibilities of the health promotion paradigm in the prevention of mental disorders.

It should be noted that the general health paradigm has an unusual and provocative solution to the question, How many different psychiatric disorders are there? The first edition of the *Diagnostic and Statistical Manual of Mental Disorders* (43) suggested that the answer was 60, the second edition (44) suggested it was 145, and the third edition (45) suggests that the answer is 230. The health promotion paradigm suggests the answer is one. To put the health promotion paradigm into the form of a testable hypothesis would be to suggest that the variance in human behavior that is accounted for by a simple assessment of degree of misery, demoralization (46), or nonspecific psychological distress (47) is significantly greater than that accounted for by any specific disorder. Testing this hypothesis may be one of the most important research agendas for the next decade.

Some uncertainty exists about how to define mental disorders in the context of primary prevention. One hears, for example, that the inability to cope with stress, the presence of an existential dilemma, feelings of unhappiness, or pathological interpersonal relationships are not real mental disorders, and thus efforts to prevent those conditions are not credible. Yet few mental health professionals will not consider treating a prospective patient who complains of the inability to cope with stress, a pervasive sense of meaninglessness in life, or a chronic inability to establish satisfying long-lasting relationships. I urge practitioners who are considering how to identify a mental disorder worthy of being prevented to adopt a general principle: If it is a condition that mental health professionals would treat, then it is a condition that we have an equal responsibility to try to prevent.

Seven years ago, the President's Commission on Mental Health completed its final report (48). The recommendations of that illustrious and far-sighted group on the subject of prevention were appropriate, timely, and prudent:

1. Establishment of a Center for Prevention within the National Institute of Mental Health (NIMH),
2. Development of special programs directed toward children at risk,
3. The creation of services and programs oriented around times of significant life stress, and
4. The expenditure of 10 percent of the NIMH budget on studies pertinent to the prevention of mental disorders.

Implementation of these efforts has already begun, and the continued active support of all mental health professionals is merited.

To wait until all direct treatment needs are met before significant resources are devoted to prevention efforts will doom our professions to the hopeless spiral we have been facing for generations. Every time NIMH funds a study of the prevalence of mental disorder in the United States, the results are more melancholy than the last time. From the 20 million mentally ill persons during the post-World War II era, we succeeded in climbing to 30 million mentally ill in the late 1970s, to the estimated 40 million mentally ill today (49).

In order to extend our knowledge base in the field of primary prevention, money will have to continue to be diverted from direct treatment programs. During 1980, the direct cost of mental health care was reported to be more than 30 billion dollars; if indirect costs due to lost productivity were included, this figure would be even higher (50). In terms of the total cost of mental illness to our society, diversion of resources from treatment to prevention research not only is little to ask but, more important, represents the only hope we have for the ultimate control of mental disorders.

REFERENCES

1. Gruenberg EM: Mental disorders, in Maxcy-Rosenau Public Health and Preventive Medicine (11th edition). Edited by Last JM. New York, Appleton-Century-Crofts, 1980
2. Gruenberg EM: The failures of success. Milbank Memorial Fund Quarterly 55:3-24, 1977
3. Adam CT: A descriptive definition of primary prevention. Journal of Primary Prevention 2:67-79, 1981
4. Perlmutter FD, Vayda AM, Woodburn PK: An instrument for differentiating programs in prevention--primary, secondary, and tertiary. Am J Orthopsychiatry 46:533-541, 1976
5. Dubos R: Mirage of Health: Utopias, Progress, and Biological Change. New York, Harper, 1959
6. Engel GL: The need for a new medical model: a challenge for biomedicine. Science 196:129-136, 1977
7. Engel GL: The clinical application of the biopsychosocial model. Am J Psychiatry 137:535-544, 1980
8. Engel GL: The biopsychosocial model: extending the scope of scientific medicine, in Critical Issues in Behavioral Medicine. Edited by West LJ, Stein M. Philadelphia, Lippincott, 1982
9. Mirsky IA: The psychosomatic approach to the etiology of clinical disorders. Psychosom Med 19:424-430, 1957
10. Eastwood MR: The Relation Between Physical and Mental Illness. Toronto, University of Toronto Press, 1975
11. Hankin J, Oktay, JS: Mental Disorder and Primary Medical Care: An Analytical Review of the Literature (DHEW Publication No. ADM 78-661). Washington, DC, U.S. Government Printing Office, 1979
12. Kellner R: Psychiatric ill health following physical illness. Br J Psychiatry 112:71-73, 1966
13. Regier DA, Shapiro S, Kessler LG, et al: Epidemiology and health service resource allocation policy for alcohol, drug abuse, and mental disorders. Public Health Rep 99:483-492, 1984
14. Taube CA, Burns BJ, Kessler L: Patients of psychiatrists and psychologists in office-based practice: 1980. Am Psychol 39:1435-1447, 1984
15. Ware JE, Manning WG, Duan N, et al: Health status and the use of outpatient mental health services. Am Psychol 39:1090-1100, 1984
16. Dumont MP: The nonspecificity of mental illness. Am J Orthopsychiatry 54:326-334, 1984
17. Rabkin JG: Stressful life events and schizophrenia: a review of the research literature. Pscyhol Bull 87:408-425, 1980

18. Brown GW, Harris T: Social Origins of Depression: A Study of Psychiatric Disorders in Women. New York, Free Press, 1978
19. Hudgens RW, Morrison JR, Barcha RG: Life events and onset of primary affective disorders. Arch Gen Psychiatry 16:134-145, 1967
20. Bloom BL, Asher SJ, White SW: Marital disruption as a stressor: a review and analysis. Psychol Bull 85:867-894, 1978
21. Bloom BL: Stressful Life Event Theory and Research: Implications for Primary Prevention (DHHS Publication No. ADM 85-1385). Washington, DC, U.S. Government Printing Office, 1985
22. Cohen F: Personality, stress, and the development of physical illness, in Health Psychology: A Handbook. Edited by Stone GC, Cohen F, Adler NE. San Francisco, CA, Jossey-Bass, 1979
23. Hinkle LE: The effect of exposure to cultural change, social change, and changes in interpersonal relationships on health, in Stressful Life Events: Their Nature and Effects. Edited by Dohrenwend BS, Dohrenwend BS. New York, Wiley, 1974
24. Aakster CW: Psychosocial stress and health disturbances. Soc Sci Med 8:77-90, 1974
25. Gallin RS: Life difficulties, coping, and the use of medical services. Cult Med Psychiatry 4:249-269, 1980
26. Cooke DJ, Greene JG: Types of life events in relation to symptoms at the climacterium. J Psychosom Res 25:5-11, 1981
27. Totman R: What makes life events stressful: a retrospective study of patients who have suffered a first myocardial infarction. J Psychosom Res 23:193-201, 1979
28. Rowland KF: Environmental events predicting death for the elderly. Psychol Bull 84:349-372, 1977
29. Sarason SB: The Psychological Sense of Community: prospects for a Community Psychology. San Francisco, Jossey-Bass, 1974
30. Bandura A: Self-efficacy: Toward a unifying theory of behavioral change. Psychol Rev 84:191-215, 1977
31. Rappaport J: In praise of paradox: a social policy of empowerment over prevention. Am J Community Psychol 9:1-21, 1981
32. Spivack G, Shure MB: Social Adjustment of Young Children: A Cognitive Approach to Solving Real-Life Problems. San Francisco, Jossey-Bass, 1973
33. Shure MB, Spivack G: Interpersonal problem-solving in young children: a cognitive approach to prevention. Am J Community Psychol 10:341-356, 1982
34. Lalonde M: A New Perspective on the Health of Canadians. Ottawa, Canadian Government Printing Office, 1974
35. Albee GW: The answer is prevention. Psychology Today, February 1985, 60-64

36. U.S. Department of Health and Human Services: Bibliography on Smoking and Health: 1983 (DHHS Publication No. PHS 84-50196). Washington, DC, U.S. Government Printing Office, 1984
37. Russell MAH, Wilson C, Taylor C, et al: Effect of general practitioners' advice against smoking. Br Med J 2:231-235, 1979
38. McPheeters HL: Primary prevention and health promotion in mental health. Prev Med 5:187-198, 1976
39. Bloom BL, Hodges WF, Kern MB, et al: A preventive intervention program for the newly separated: final evaluations. Am J Orthopsychiatry 55:9-26, 1985
40. Felner RD, Ginter M, Primavera J: Primary prevention during school transitions: social support and environmental structure. Am J Community Psychol 10:227-290, 1982
41. Lynch JJ: The Language of the Heart: The Body's Response to Human Dialogue. New York, Basic Books, 1985
42. Melamed BG, Bush JP: Maternal-child influences during medical procedures, in Issues in Clinical and Community Psychology: Crisis Intervention With Children and Families. Edited by Auerbach SM, Stolberg AL. New York, Hemisphere, in press
43. American Psychiatric Association: Diagnostic and Statistical Manual of Mental Disorders (First Edition). Washington, DC, American Psychiatric Association, 1952
44. American Psychiatric Association: Diagnostic and Statistical Manual of Mental Disorders (Second Edition). Washington, DC, American Psychiatric Association, 1968
45. American Psychiatric Association: Diagnostic and Statistical Manual of Mental Disorders (Third Edition). Washington, DC, American Psychiatric Association, 1980
46. Frank JD: Persuasion and Healing. Baltimore, MD, Johns Hopkins University Press, 1973
47. Dohrenwend BP, Shrout PE, Egri G, et al: Nonspecific psychological distress and other dimensions of psychopathology: measures for use in the general population. Arch Gen Psychiatry 37:1229-1236, 1980
48. President's Commission on Mental Health: Report to the President. Washington, DC, U.S. Government Printing Office, 1978
49. Robins LN, Helzer JE, Weissman MM, et al: Lifetime prevalence of specific psychiatric disorders in three sites. Arch Gen Psychiatry 41:949-958, 1984
50. American Psychiatric Association: Economic Fact Book for Psychiatry. Washington, DC, American Psychiatric Association, 1983

2

Cross-Cultural Perspectives on Primary Prevention of Mental Disorders

Ricardo F. Muñoz, Ph.D.

Florentius Chan, Ph.D.

Regina Armas, Ph.D.

2

Cross-Cultural Perspectives on Prevention: Primary Prevention of Mental Disorders

The goal of primary prevention is to forestall unnecessary human suffering. In addition, it may reduce direct treatment costs as well as indirect costs to society such as for physical health care due to mental disorders, reduced job productivity, and family disruption. In this chapter, primary prevention concepts are examined from a cross-cultural perspective, reports of prevention work with four specific cultural groups are reviewed, and directions for future work are suggested.

CROSS-CULTURAL PERSPECTIVES ON MENTAL HEALTH

Marsella (1) divided the concerns of cross-cultural psychiatry into four basic questions:

1. Is there a universal concept of "normal" and abnormal" behavior?
2. Are there differences in the rates of mental disorders across cultures?
3. Are there differences in the manifestations or patterns of mental disorders across cultures?
4. Are there relationships between the sociocultural milieu and various aspects of mental disorders?

These questions are important because they raise issues regarding the target of preventive interventions across cultures, the universality of our diagnostic frameworks, and the possible influences that each culture has on the mental health of its members and others. In addition to these questions, those of us interested in primary prevention must ask whether preventive interventions are likely to be uniformly effective across cultures, and, if not, how they ought to be adapted to specific groups.

Increasing the difficulty in determining whether at least some portion of mental disorders are significantly influenced by cultural factors is the fact that most psychiatric services and mental health research studies available in other countries are characterized by an imposition of Western standards (1, 2). Diagnostic schemes used by Western-trained professionals may force manifestations of pathology into clusters that may or may not be helpful in understanding how to best intervene or prevent them. The effect of imported settings, such as the mental hospital, may shape patients' behavior toward stereotypy and uniformity (3).

Substantial variations in rates of mental disorders from country to country have been reported, but methodological differences across studies make comparisons between them problematic (4). The expression of mental disorders also has been documented to vary across cultures. For example, there are cultures that do not have terms equivalent to *depression* (5). Relationships between culture and mental disorders have been hypothesized to occur because of differing cultural practices. For example, in the case of depression, Marsella (1) speculated that practices such as multiple mothering and the role of the extended family may reduce the impact of parent loss, the widespread use of projection as a defense mechanism may reduce the prevalence of self-blame in depressives, and practices such as mourning rituals and ancestor worship may reduce the impact of losing loved ones.

Although the controversy about the relative impact of culture on psychopathology is far from resolved, contemporary opinions regarding certain aspects of the controversy favor certain conclusions (6). The more common Western diagnostic categories are presumed to have universal applicability. Differences in rates of mental disorders across countries are believed to be due primarily to differences in the diagnostic criteria used. The expression of symptoms (such as the nature of delusions and hallucinations) are expected to be culturally determined, at least to some degree. A number of recognizable syndromes (amok, susto, and the current common eating disorders in the United States) are known to occur within certain temporal, geographical, and cultural boundaries.

Other areas are much more heatedly discussed, such as the nature of the known relationship between the socioeconomic environment and mental disorders. Two views on this are social causation theory and social selection theory. The former holds that the level of psychopathology is a function of the amount of adversity and stress produced by the social environment. The latter holds that differential rates of psychopathology are due to the downward drift of dysfunctional individuals. An impressive attempt to decide which theory is best supported by available epidemiologic data was made by the Dohrenwends (7), who concluded that social causation appears to better explain the rate patterns of schizophrenia, delinquency, antisocial personality, and problem drinking.

Because the cross-cultural literature on mental health is so extensive and filled with many intricate controversies, this chapter focuses on four minority groups in the United States: American Indians, Asians, Blacks, and Hispanics. These groups are significantly overrepresented in the lower socioeconomic classes, which means that large proportions of their members are at high risk for psychological problems. The clearest findings in the epidemiological literature are that inverse relationships exist between social class and the prevalence of schizophrenia, personality disorders, and nonspecific psychological distress (7). There may also be an inverse relationship between social class and unipolar affective disorder, although this is not as clear and may be limited to women with children (7-9). (Interestingly, bipolar disorder may be relatively less prevalent in lower socioeconomic groups.)

Within each of these four groups--American Indians, Asians, Blacks, and Hispanics--a great diversity of cultures exists. In this chapter they are grouped into the four categories to simplify the presentation.

PRIMARY PREVENTION AND MINORITY GROUPS IN THE UNITED STATES

Among the many reasons given for the need for preventive services in the four identified minority groups in the United States is the relative poverty in which many of their members live. The role of the socioeconomic environment on health status was identified clearly in *Healthy People: The Surgeon General's Report on Health Promotion and Disease Prevention* (10). The poor face greater health risks than do people in higher income groups, such as inadequate medical care with too few preventive services; more hazardous physical environment, greater risk for violence or homicide; less education; more unemployment or unsatisfying job experiences; and income inadequate for good nutrition, safe housing, and other basic needs (10).

In *Health and Behavior: Frontiers of Research in the Biobehavioral Sciences*, a report by the National Academy of Sciences

Institute of Medicine (11), evidence is reviewed on the higher rates of death and disability in poor populations. It is pointed out that "even when causative factors of a disease are unknown and treatments are unavailable, changes in socioeconomic conditions and literacy rates can reduce mortality. One example of this phenomenon is the decline in mortality from tuberculosis before the availability of chemotherapy" (p. 215). It is further pointed out that most of the differences found in health status between minorities and Whites become negligible when studies are controlled for social class.

The need to control for social class in epidemiological studies is important because of the danger of attributing differences in health, productivity, and social success to race or ethnicity. Such attributions can be used to support racist or ethnocentric beliefs of genetic or cultural superiority. On the other hand, it is important to remember that when we control for social class and differences in health risk disappear, they are disappearing only statistically. Given the distribution of income across ethnic groups in the United States, if socioeconomic status is related to higher risk, then minority groups are more likely to be at greater risk and ought to continue receiving great attention in terms of preventive efforts. For example, minority death rates in the United States exceed White death rates in all age groups up to age 80 (11). Health service availability to the poor will not by itself change this state of affairs. For example, even with their major efforts to make health services available to the poor, Great Britain continues to experience these differentials (12).

The long-term effects of health and socioeconomic differences between White and minority groups are likely to have negative effects on both groups. To illustrate how a cross-cultural perspective can bring out important information that is otherwise ignored, let us examine a specific example in detail.

David Hayes-Bautista (13) brought to our attention the changing shape of population pyramids for the many ethnic groups in California and the effects these demographic changes may have. Because of their possible impact on stress levels on all the cultural groups involved, it is worthwhile to consider his observations.

In a population pyramid, rectangular blocks representing age brackets lie one on top of the other. Usually the length of the bottom block represents the number of children from 0 to 10 years of age, the length of one immediately above it represents the number of individuals 11 to 20 years of age, and so on. Because of high numbers of children and relatively high death rates across the entire age span, population blocks traditionally become shorter as age increases. Thus their pyramidal shape.

However, as Dr. John Talbott pointed out in an address entitled "Social Issues and Decisions That Will Effect Change in the Practice of Psychiatry" at the 1985 annual meeting of the American Psychiatric Association (14), population pyramids for the United States no longer look like pyramids. They are rectangular in shape, with each age bracket having approximately the same number of individuals. This state of affairs is a major sign of the great advances that the United States has made in terms of providing the majority of its population with a better standard of living and the type of preventive health care that has reduced premature mortality. Talbott's comments focused on how the dynamics of demographics, economics, service delivery, and regulation influence the practice of psychiatry today and will shape its future. As the proportion of persons over age 65 becomes larger and larger in the United States's population, at some point in the not too distant future those who are still in the work force will be supporting retirees equal to them in numbers. Given that the work force is already showing an unwillingness to increase their support for social security and other aid to the aged, a number of difficult questions are raised.

Hayes-Bautista examined cross-cultural influences in the composition of the United States population. His first interesting finding was that the cultural/ethnic groups in California that are presently referred to as "minorities" do have population pyramids that are pyramidally shaped. Among other reasons, this is because they have more children and they die younger. Whites in California, as in the rest of the United States, have more rectangular pyramids. As one projects these pyramids into the early 21st century, one finds that the majority of the working force in California will be composed of Hispanics, Blacks, and Asians and that the over age 65 group will be predominantly White. This cross-cultural perspective allows us to see that not only will we have a gradually smaller work force supporting a gradually larger number of older persons, but we will also have a predominantly non-White work force supporting a predominantly White aged population.

There are many implications to these demographic trends:

- If present educational and wage level differences continue, the minority work force will have relatively low-paying jobs and will find it difficult to make a comfortable living, let alone support a large group of retirees.
- If present tensions across racial and ethnic groups continue, we will find a reversal of the present feeling of anger from White wage earners who do not want their money to be used to support social programs for poor, largely non-White groups to

resentment from non-White wage earners asked to support an aged White population.

- The epidemiology of psychiatric disorders will show major changes as age-related disorders become confounded with race and ethnicity. For example, Alzheimer's disease will be more prevalent in the White population, simply because that group will be older. New cases of schizophrenia will come predominantly from the younger non-White groups.
- Social support differences across cultural groups will have greater impact on health status. For example, Whites may be less likely than non-Whites to obtain familial support during old age given their cultural preference for inculcating independence and encouraging geographical mobility, especially for career building. This will increase high-risk factors such as increased loneliness and its sequelae (15) and will reduce protective factors such as available support systems (for example, the family), which have served us well for most of our evolutionary history.
- The confounding of age with ethnicity will mirror the present confounding of social class with ethnicity and may produce negative prejudices toward the older Whites, who will be seen as absorbing social resources and not contributing to the production of wealth.

It is important to try to avert a possible source of tension in the near future as White cultural groups become more at risk than they are now. For example, we could focus attention on actively increasing the earning potential of those groups who will bear the brunt of supporting the older population. We could accelerate efforts to make available the advances made in the United States in living standards and preventive health care to the non-White groups so that their population pyramids begin to resemble those of the White groups, thus reducing the differential relationship between age and race. We could consider methods to promote greater affection and respect among the many cultural and ethnic groups in the United States population. Racism must be reduced in intensity and replaced with a sense of the unity of human beings in this small planet in order to avoid race-based neglect of those who are in need of assistance.

A focus on cross-cultural issues related to American Indians, Asians, Blacks, and Hispanics in the United States is important because these groups compose approximately 16.9 percent of the United States population (16). There is evidence that patterns of utilization of clinical services for minorities are different from those of whites. Retention and outcome may also differ: Prevention services might be more acceptable to minorities. Cross-cultural comparisons within one country may test the limits of and the extent to which we can generalize our mental health concepts without the confounding effects of different availability of mental health resources across countries. Finally, studying cultural factors that reduce incidence of mental disorders within each group may provide us with hypotheses and prevention intervention ideas that could be used in the other groups.

Prevention Services

We suspect that many prevention programs that serve multiethnic populations have not been documented in the literature. Out of 1,008 references in an annotated bibliography on primary prevention in mental health published in 1985, 11 references focused on American Indians, 11 on Blacks, 8 on Hispanics, and 1 on Asians (17). Most of the references reported suggestions for preventive work, rather than presenting completed or ongoing preventive programs.

We will discuss successively those programs offering preventive services to American Indians, Asians, Blacks, and Hispanics. If a program serves more than one group, it will be included in the discussion of the group most heavily represented. Unfortunately, many programs intended to be preventive have little or no evaluation component built in. Thus, we are unable to judge their effect. (In fairness to these programs, we should point out that most treatment services are not evaluated either).

Prevention Research

Very few prevention research studies are designed explicitly to obtain representation from each of the major minority groups. In this section, we describe a study currently being conducted by a team of which we are part.

The San Francisco Depression Prevention Research Project is a randomized controlled prevention trial supported in part by the National Institute of Mental Health (NIMH; 18). Its goal is to develop and evaluate a cognitive-behavioral intervention designed to reduce the incidence of clinical depression (major depression and dysthymia) in medical outpatients, with a special emphasis on low-income minority users of public primary care clinics. Since the study is being conducted in San Francisco, which is 22 percent Asian, 12 percent Hispanic, and 12 percent Black, it was considered necessary to make sure that we included in the sample significant numbers of these cultural groups. In fact, since minorities are overrepresented in most of the clinics studied, the proportion of minorities should have been even greater than for the city as a whole.

The study consists of two parts: a) a comprehensive screening and assessment procedure and b) the randomized trial itself. More than 10,000 medical patients were prescreened for the preliminary inclusion criteria, which included having an open chart for six months or more and being between 18 and 69 years of age. Of these, 3,859 patients were contacted either by letter or when they came to the clinics for a medical appointment. Individuals were asked if they would be willing to participate in a year-long research study that would require six two-hour interviews and random assignment to one of two conditions (one of which would require attendance at a class meeting two hours a week for eight weeks). Five hundred and forty-eight people agreed and entered the screening part of the project.

The screening included administration of the NIMH Diagnostic Interview Schedule (19, 20) plus 16 other measures that assess factors such as social supports, life events, health service utilization, quality of life ratings, and cognitive-behavioral variables (activity level, thinking patterns, social activities, and so on). Persons who met criteria in the *Diagnostic and Statistical Manual of Mental Disorders (Third Edition) (DSM-III; 21)* for major depression or other major disorders (for example, schizophrenia, current drug abuse) or who were already receiving mental health treatment were not included in the study and, if appropriate, were referred for treatment. Thus the final sample was a true primary prevention sample. Participants who repeatedly missed screening appointments were also deleted in order to increase the chances that those who entered the randomized part of the study would follow through with the periodic follow-up interviews. Those who completed initial interviews and met all criteria for inclusion were randomly assigned to the experimental or control conditions. The sample in the randomized trial consists of 175 individuals, 36 percent of whom are White, 19 percent Black, 22 percent Hispanic, and 23 percent Asian. It is important to note that we would not have obtained such a large non-White population had we not provided language-appropriate screening and intervention. In the Hispanic group, 74 percent are completing the study in Spanish. In the Asian group, 63 percent are completing the study in Chinese (Cantonese and Mandarin). All measures and intervention protocols were translated into Spanish and Chinese by using the forward-backward translation method. They were then reviewed by bilingual and bicultural staff. Examples and concepts were rewritten when necessary to make them more culturally appropriate.

The intervention is a course entailing eight weekly two-hour classes that presents a number of cognitive-behavioral techniques found to be effective in the treatment of nonbipolar depression (22). Each session covers the rationale for the self-control techniques, exercises designed to individualize the methods, and homework to facilitate use of the methods in daily situations.

The study is still in progress. The results will be used to estimate incidence of clinical depression in this population and effect size of the intervention in terms of differential number of new cases in each of the groups. We will also examine effect size on depression symptom scales, quality of life, and medical utilization. An important analysis will focus on the effects of the intervention on the hypothesized cognitive-behavioral mediating variables, which are the proximal target of the intervention and are theorized to produce the preventive effect. The psychometric properties of the instruments across the ethnic groups will also be examined.

PRIMARY PREVENTION AND AMERICAN INDIANS

The American Indian population consists of dozens of nations or tribes among which vast differences exist in language, culture, and philosophy. Including Alaska natives and Aleuts, American Indians currently comprise 0.6 percent of the United States population (16). There is a paucity of studies that focus on prevalence of psychiatric disorders among American Indians. Manson et al. (23) indicated that only three epidemiological studies have been carried out on a community-wide basis. Shore et al. (24) assessed approximately half of the adult population in a Pacific northwest coast village. Roy et al. (25) surveyed approximately 25 percent of the total Indian population of 10 reservations, and Sampath (26) interviewed 93 percent of the population of an Eskimo settlement. Estimated prevalence of psychiatric disorders in these communities was extremely high, ranging from 27 percent (25) to 54 percent (24). Moreover, both Roy et al. and Shore et al. found that confirmed cases were more common among younger people than among their older counterparts. For example, in the Roy et al. study, one-third of the active cases were composed of children, 63 percent of whom were suffering from various *DSM-II* classifications of neurosis. For a thorough overview of primary, secondary, and tertiary research on problems such as alcoholism, drug abuse, child abuse and neglect, mental retardation, suicide, and other major and minor psychiatric disorders in the American Indian population, we recommend Manson et al.'s review (23).

The literature suggests that American Indians do use mental health services (27), particularly when these services are delivered in culturally appropriate ways (28). In fact, use of mental health services among American Indians has increased in recent years (29).

However, there continue to be too few culturally appropriate mental health services available to meet the needs of the American Indian population. Many services are inaccessible to the general population and/or are delivered by therapists or counselors who are insensitive to Indian world views (30, 31).

One major reason for the low level of use of mental health services may be related to the lack of Indian professionals. Trimble (32) estimated that only approximately 70 American Indians have doctoral degrees in the fields of anthropology, psychiatry, psychology, social work, or sociology. Moreover, Trimble noted, only a few of these professionals work in areas that directly affect American Indian populations.

Prevention Services

There is documentation that in recent years a handful of culturally relevant prevention services have been developed for American Indians. Preventive services have focused on mental health promotion for children and their families (33-35); on specific problems, such as alcohol abuse (36, 37); or on improving the social environment in culturally specific ways (38, 39).

Focusing on preventive services for children, Shore et al. (34) reported on an Indian-sponsored group home for children and adolescents, designed to limit off-reservation foster and adoption placements. A number of mental health and social services were made available to the residents. By reviewing various record systems, the authors determined that 20 percent of the youth population had off-reservation placements prior to the establishment of the home; this dropped to less than 1 percent once the group home was operating. Looking at two time periods, 1974 and 1979, Shore et al. compared demographic variables through a random selection of 10 charts per time period. The reasons for group home referral were found to change over time from primarily child abuse/neglect cases to ones of adolescent misbehavior. No data are available to clearly explain why the reasons for placements changed. One possible explanation, noted by the authors, is that by 1979 most of the children who needed child abuse/neglect protection services had been served and the older children were referred to a treatment facility.

Red Horse (33) reported on a natural support network program for high school students, using the Indian concept of the family as the treatment model. The program helped students establish new network ties or recognize dysfunctional ones by identifying behavioral expectations in the network. Although no evaluative data were provided, the author noted that "school attendance, performance, and family relationship of participants improved over the course of their involvement in the program; the frequency of their encounters with the juvenile system decreased markedly" (33, p. 182).

Haven et al. (37) reported on 14 distinct community prevention projects of the United Southern and Easter Tribes, of which the major focus was on alcoholism. Kleinfeld (38) reported on two settings wherein providing a positive socializing environment developed competencies in Eskimo youth who were at high risk for social dysfunction.

Prevention Research

One of the few prevention trials in mental health promotion for American Indians was carried out by Dinges (40). This study focused on the relationship between young Navajo children (infants to four-year-olds) and their parents. The intervention consisted of home visits designed to promote cultural identification, strengthen family ties, and enhance the self-image of the child and parent.

In Dinges's study, a culturally relevant intervention was conscientiously developed and implemented. First, the project was carried out from a transcultural perspective, that is, on the assumption that "it is possible for persons from a minority culture to acquire the skills, knowledge, and material lifestyle of a majority culture, without sacrificing the identity-supporting elements of the minority culture" (40, p. 123). Dinges acknowledges that his viewpoint is controversial. It has been criticized by those who believe that exposure to values of the dominant society leads to deterioration of cultural functioning.

Second, to avoid the possibility of culturally inappropriate interventions, the researchers a) explicitly considered the Navajo beliefs about psychosocial development, the causes of life and of individual behavior; b) conducted a survey to determine current child-rearing beliefs and practices, thereby generating active community involvement; and c) used a conceptual model that allowed for cultural variations in individuals and their families (that is, they did not take a static view of culturally appropriate responses).

This outcome study used a post-test-only design with a matched comparison group. To minimize problems in collecting measures from the comparison group, Dinges a) established rapport with these families before assessment interviews took place, b) arranged a "mini-project experience" for these families after all data were collected, and (c) obtained widespread community acceptance of the project, which facilitated comparison families' interest.

Finally, Dinges's research team addressed the lack of culturally appropriate mental health measures by adapting existing measures to make them more culturally applicable. Moreover, they relied heavily on observational methods (including videotaping) to compile needed data.

Recruitment was by self-selection, after announcements were made in the community. Eventually, 57 families were assigned to the intervention condition and 54 to the comparison group.

The outcome data of the study are described in detail by Dinges (40). The intervention families reported fewer depressive symptoms, fewer psychosomatic symptoms, and less feeling of isolation and loneliness.

Other randomized trials have focused on specific problems common to American Indian communities. For example, Carpenter et al. (36) conducted a pilot evaluation study that focused on prevention of alcohol abuse in American Indian high school students. Thirty students, who had been identified as having emerging drinking problems, were selected to participate in a secondary prevention intervention in which peer-mediated self-control training was provided.

Three interventions were made available: 1) an 11-week alcohol education class dealing with information on controlled social drinking, 2) self-control information sessions, and 3) self-monitoring. Students were randomly assigned to one of three conditions. Group A received all three interventions, Group B received self-control sessions and self-monitoring, and Group C received self-monitoring only. All three groups met with a peer counselor three times a week.

All groups significantly decreased the quantity and frequency of weekly alcohol consumption, a change that was maintained over 12 months. The authors noted limitations of the data, in that the number of study participants was small, they relied heavily on self-report data, and they did not incorporate a no-treatment group. Nevertheless, Carpenter et al. note, the findings parallel those of other studies in which little or no differences were found between extensive and minimal interventions, as long as both included self-monitoring and self-help guidelines.

An example of a culture-specific preventive research project is the Tiospaye project (39). "Tiospaye" is a Sioux word that describes a community way of life that is patterned by Lakota Sioux rules for social interactions, rituals for transition, identity acquisition, healing, and by a set of values.

Sioux leaders considered this way of life healthy and wished to explore it as a method for preventing serious psychological and social pathology. The exploration procedure entailed 1) assessing how traditional the community was by using ratings from community experts, 2) assessing pathology by using legal and medical indexes, and 3) then assessing the relationship between pathology and traditional status.

A "Tiospaye scale" was developed by selecting descriptive statements from community leaders and factor analyzing the items. The resulting scale yielded high interrater and test-retest reliability. In assessing pathology, they found that adult males, particularly those unemployed, were overrepresented in the medical data. In analyzing the legal data, they found that high rates of crime arrests occurred with high employment of women, active community involvement by women in conjunction with low level of involvement by older men, and high unemployment among men.

On the basis of these findings, Mohatt and Blue implemented a community intervention at one of four available communities. The intervention consisted of meeting with community residents to identify community needs and working with the residents on three identified activities: economic projects, construction of a hall, and promotion of health and social activities. Results showed that the intervention did not improve the Tiospaye scores for the targeted community; in fact, they decreased slightly. However, the other three communities showed a marked decrease in Tiospaye scores. The intervention did not significantly alter measurable pathology in the community.

Recently, other randomized preventive trials have been initiated. For example, Manson (41) and his associates have begun a randomized, controlled intervention designed to prevent depression in older American Indians suffering from poor physical health. This study is taking place in three reservation communities and is the first culture-specific intervention trial of its kind.

Another example is Mamak's (42) use of a randomized control design to implement a community-based intervention program for high-risk, middle-aged American Samoan men. The goal of the study is to promote community and social competence, while assisting high-risk individuals to develop a self-reliant coping strategy. It is hypothesized that these two factors will prevent or reduce symptoms in various psychiatric disorders. The study is designed to accommodate 285 males who are free from any major psychopathology. One hundred and ninety subjects will be randomly assigned to an experimental group and 95 subjects to a control condition. The project plans to use community leaders (paraprofessionals) as "change agents" to deliver a six-month intervention that uses an educational strategy designed to develop personal and social coping skills. Regular follow-up assessments for 18 months after intervention are planned.

PRIMARY PEVENTION AND ASIANS

Asian Americans demonstrated rapid population growth in the last decade, primarily because of a large influx of Asian immigrants and refugees. Around 700,000 refugees have come from Southeast Asia since 1975 (43). Although the admission rates of Asian Americans to mental health services have significantly increased in recent years, they still reflect underutilization (44, 45).

There are many reasons for the underutilization of mental health services (46). Two are the different belief systems about mental health and the stigma associated with mental illness. Non-Westernized Asian Americans often attribute the development of mental illness to organic factors (for example, imbalance between yin and yang, "weak" liver) and supernatural factors (for example, demonic possession, retribution for a sin) rather than to psychological factors (47). Even if they consider specific problems to be psychological, they are very reluctant to use mental health services because of the strong social stigma involved (46). Such reluctance results in longer delay in seeking help (48), greater severity of mental disturbance by the time they finally seek help (49), or inappropriate medical treatment (50).

Compared with treatment, primary prevention has been argued to be more acceptable to Asian Americans. First, primary prevention, with its emphasis on promotion of mental health, could avoid the stigma associated with mental illness. Second, since primary prevention is usually based on a community model or a psychoeducational approach, it matches well the conceptualization of mental health in this population (50).

Prevention Services

Many prevention programs with Asian Americans have been established in recent years (52). Although the target population (for example, children or the elderly) and the formats (for example, mass media or the classroom) are different, they share an emphasis on promotion of well-being or health rather than on prevention of a specific mental illness. This emphasis fits well with the Asian belief that disease prevention and health promotion are part of the same process (53). Strong well-being that includes good health and will power is believed to be essential in mastering difficulties and preventing illness (47).

Immigrant and refugee children and adolescents, compared with adults, are more vulnerable to psychological problems because they find themselves caught between two cultures (54). Helping both the children and their parents to identify the risk factors for these conflicts could prevent children from developing various types of psychological problems.

Because of the influx of immigrants and refugees in the last decade, many volunteer agencies (for example, voluntary resettlement agency or newcomer service) have been established to expedite resettlement. Among these agencies, the Mutual Assistance Association has the longest history and the greatest number of clients. Since 1975, close to 1,000 Mutual Assistance Associations have emerged from within the Asian community throughout this country (55). The purposes and orientations of these associations are diverse. However, after studying these associations for more than 10 years, Khoa and Bui (56) concluded that they share one or more of five major focuses. These focuses are cultural and spiritual integrity, resettlement service provision, advocacy, and political action, special shared interests, and economic development. Although there is no formal evaluation of the services provided by these associations, it is believed that they promote a sense of identity, increase social support networks, and enhance adaptation skills.

Prevention Research

One of the early prevention studies on identity conflicts was performed by Yee and Lee (53). These authors developed a primary prevention program with Filipino youths in a high school. The purposes of the program were to provide the participants with a positive view of their cultural identity and a supportive environment in which to examine how their cultural values and behaviors differ from those of other Americans. Participants were 45 tenth- to twelfth-grade students from two Filipino bilingual-bicultural classes. The program consisted of 10 weekly sessions of 50 minutes each. It focused on four general areas, namely, basic communication skills, self and identity, self and society, and generational values. The evaluation of the program was limited to feedback from the participants in an interview with hired student interviewers. Results indicate that the participants obtained new knowledge about their identity, family, and values; they felt that the program should be continued.

Many of the prevention services discussed earlier are well established and have large number of participants (for example, the Mutual Assistance Association). They offer the opportunity to build in prevention research projects. One such organization integrates research with service. This is On Lok Senior Health Services in San Francisco. It is a well-organized health service for Asian elderly (56). On Lok provides a full range of medical, social, and supportive services, including day care and housing, to people who are 55 years of age and older. Approximately 75 percent of the clients are Chinese and their mean age is 78 (57). A major purpose of this organization is to promote a better quality of life that includes good physical and mental health.

A research department was established within On Lok to develop special programs and evaluate the services regularly. For example, a project entitled the Community Care Organization for Dependent Adults was developed to evaluate the impact of such a program on the quality and cost of long-term care and the health and welfare of the program participants (57). There were 496 program participants and 70 nonprogram participants in the study. Three research approaches were used simultaneously to evaluate the service: 1) process analysis, which is a qualitative analysis to describe and interpret issues in program and systems development; 2) within-group analysis, to specify the participant and mediating variables related to the outcome; and 3) comparison group analysis, based on a subset of 70 program participants and 70 nonprogram participants, to evaluate the effectiveness of the program. The findings suggested that the community-based care program is cost effective with respect to health care costs and promotes high levels of independence. However, the impact on quality of life and prevention of psychological problems still needs to be tested.

PRIMARY PREVENTION AND BLACKS

Blacks are the largest minority in the United States, at 11.7 percent of the population. Compared with Whites, Blacks are more likely to be misdiagnosed (58), overmedicated (59), seen by nonprofessionals (60), and given inappropriate treatment (61). Premature termination of psychotherapy is one reflection of this differential treatment. Sue et al. (62) found that 52.1 percent of Black patients dropped out of psychotherapy after the initial session, compared with only 29.8 percent of White patients.

Despite receiving differential treatment, Blacks tend to use mental health service more frequently than do Whites (60). In a study of 17 community mental health centers in the greater Seattle area over a three-year period, Sue (60) found that Black and American Indian patients were overrepresented by a factor of two (based on their proportion in the population), whereas Asian and Chicano patients were markedly underrepresented.

Because of racial discrimination and poverty, it is believed that Blacks experience higher levels of stress than do Whites. Many epidemiologic studies using depression symptom scales (for example, the Center for Epidemiological Studies Depression Scale) have shown Blacks to have higher levels of depression as reflected by high depression scores (63, 64). However, when the effects of socioeconomic variables are taken into account in the analyses, race differences diminish (65). A more complete picture of the prevalence of *DSM-III* psychiatric disorders among Blacks will be obtained in the Epidemiologic Catchment Area studies currently being coordinated by the NIMH. The preliminary findings of these studies reveal no significance differences between Blacks and Whites on prevalence of psychiatric disorders (65).

Prevention Services

Many community mental health centers have developed specific programs to prevent mental disorders among Blacks. The Hahneman Community Mental Health Center in Philadelphia is one example (67). The center is located in a city in which one-third of the population meet the poverty level and more than half of the population are Black. The goals of the prevention programs are to strengthen clients' stress coping skills, enhance their support networks, and increase the awareness of staff and policy makers on the importance of primary prevention.

In order to maximize the effects of primary prevention, it is imperative to motivate the target population to play an active role in the prevention program. Paster (68) described the primary prevention activities of the Washington Heights-West Harlem-Inwood Mental Health Council's Community Mental Health Center, which attempted to motivate the population's active participation. The catchment area is located in northwest Manhattan, and the population is 50 percent Black, 30 percent White, and 20 percent Hispanic. The center has integrated primary prevention activities into all aspects of the program, from the development of the proposal for the center to its governance and service delivery. The goals of these programs are to improve quality of life, develop support systems, and promote a sense of kinship among neighbors. The programs include leadership training, provision of crucial information, and development of personal competence through experiences in advocacy for community and self-interest. Observational evaluation revealed that these programs had encouraging results.

Community mental health centers usually serve populations of diverse cultural background. To better implement primary prevention programs targeted to their specific needs, staff should be very familiar with clients' cultural background. Because of the diverse cultural background of the community, the Jackson Memorial Community Mental Health Center in Miami, Florida developed six culturally specific teams (67). Slightly more than half of the people in this catchment area are Black and the rest of the population are Hispanic and White. Although the majority of the Blacks were born in the United States, some came from the Bahamas, Puerto Rico, and Haiti. The six culturally specific teams are the Geriatric, the Haitian, the Bahamian, the Black, the Cuban, and the Puerto Rican teams. Each team is staffed by people of the same cultural background. One major goal of these teams is to identify the needs of the clients they serve and develop culturally relevant prevention programs. These programs include peer counseling, promotion of social support networks, English lessons, and many other services. Observational evaluation suggested a reduction in hospital recidivism and improvement in neighborhood social indicators.

Prevention Research

One of the earlier preventive intervention studies was related to mental retardation. Heber et al. (69, 70) randomly assigned 40 expectant mothers with IQ scores below 75 (high risk for having retarded children) into either an intervention or a no-intervention group. Starting at three months of age, children of mothers in the intervention condition were exposed to an intensive educational program that focused primarily on language and cognitive skills. The program lasted all day, five days a week, 12 months per year for five years. The program was located in their neighborhoods and was conducted by paraprofessionals from the Black community. The mothers of this group also received education on budgeting, nutrition, and child development, with the aim of improving the environment for the children. Results revealed that children of the intervention group had significantly higher IQ scores (124 versus 94) than did the comparison group when both groups reached age five.

A prevention program with Black mothers and children was conducted by Shure and Spivack (71, 72). The purpose of this program was to teach subjects interpersonal cognitive problem-solving skills to prevent development of adjustment problems in children. Twenty mother-child pairs (mean age of children was 4.3 years) were assigned to an intervention condition, and twenty matched pairs were assigned to a no-intervention condition. The mothers of the intervention group received 10 weekly three-hour workshops in which they learned the interpersonal cognitive problem-solving skills and ways to teach their children these skills. Results showed that the training served the purpose of preventing adjustment problems, such as impulsive and inhibited behaviors.

Shure and Spivack performed a similar prevention project in day-care centers (73). This time the teachers of the centers provided the interpersonal cognitive problem-solving skills training to 113 Black children between ages four and five. Evaluation over a two-year period revealed that these children were less likely to show behavioral problems than were 106 comparable controls.

Students entering a new school usually experience increased stress and are susceptible to maladaptive changes in adjustment (74). A prevention project was developed by Felner et al. (75) to increase levels of peer and teacher support and thus to reduce the difficulties encountered during the transition. Students were randomly selected for participation in the project from among 450 students during the summer before they entered their freshman year at a large urban high school. The school population was 57 percent Black, 22 percent Hispanic, 19 percent White, and 2 percent other. The participants were 65 students who showed satisfactory school adjustment and were not in need of any special mental health program. The 65 participants of this Transition Project (the experimental group) were matched with 120 control students from the same school. The project was to restructure the role of homeroom teachers and to reduce the impact of the social setting confronting the students by reorganizing the school environment. Assessments were made at the midpoint and end of the school year. Results revealed that the experimental subjects had significantly better attendance records and grade point averages as well as self-concept than did the control subjects. The experimental subjects also perceived the school environment as having clearer expectations and organizational structure and higher levels of teacher support than did the Control subjects.

Although the aforementioned prevention projects demonstrated significant preventive effects across time (for example, two years), the evaluation was limited to performance in the same setting. It is of conceptual importance to show that preventive intervention can produce effects that generalize across time, settings, and behaviors (76). To evaluate such effects, Bry (76) performed a follow-up (at one and five years) on the subjects from the Bry and George (77, 78) studies. The subjects were 44 male and 22 female high school students. Half were randomly assigned to the intervention group; the others were assigned to the control group. Their mean age was 15.5; 42 percent were Black and 52 percent were White. They were selected into the Bry and George studies because they exhibited problems in at least two of three areas: low academic motivation, feeling of distance from family, or discipline problems. The preventive intervention, which was based on behavior modification and lasted for two years, was aimed at improving problems in the three areas. School records and interviews one year after the intervention program and arrest records at five years showed that the intervention prevented deliquency problems. These results supported their hypothesis that exposing high-risk adolescents to preventive intervention can reduce the incidence of delinquency.

A primary prevention program was designed to enhance individual and community competence in older adult community workers and in community residents with whom they worked (78). Individual competence was defined in terms of a sense of self-efficacy, a world attitude that included hope and interpersonal trust, and relevant behavioral attributes such as problem-solving skills. Similarly, community competence was defined as having alternatives and knowing how to obtain and use resources, thereby counteracting feelings of powerlessness. A sample of 22 community workers (11 Black, 10 White, 1 Hispanic) with an average age of 63 years participated in the study. They attended a two-day workshop in which they learned skills in interviewing, active listening, problem solving, and using community resources. After this workshop, they spent eight or more hours a week for two years in project activities and attended weekly meetings to review cases and continue to improve skills. A total of 97 community residents with whom these community workers worked also participated in the study. These residents were comparable to the community workers in age, race, and sex. They completed individual and community competence measures before beginning their project involvement and after one and two years of participation. At the time of the Year 1 posttest, a new random sample of 30 residents was generated that served as a posttest-only control group. The posttest results revealed increased knowledge of community services among all intervention participants, increased use of community information channels, and increased life satisfaction for the community workers. The community residents, particularly Blacks, perceived greater sense of personal control. This study demonstrated that preventive effects can be expanded by training community workers as paraprofessionals.

PRIMARY PREVENTION AND HISPANICS

The term *Hispanic* refers not to one population, but to many (80). Hispanics are the fastest growing minority in the United States.

Currently, they represent 6.4 percent of the population (16). It is assumed that the figure would be even higher if a complete census count on the undocumented Hispanics living in the United States could be obtained. Chicanos, or people of Mexican descent, represent the largest proportion of Hispanics (60 percent), followed by Puerto Ricans (14 percent), Cubans (5 percent), and other Spanish origin (21 percent). To add to the heterogeneity of the Hispanic group, some families can trace their roots in the United States back more than 300 years, while others are recent immigrants. Changes in social, political, and economic factors in Latin America directly affect immigration patterns, as evidenced by recent increases in number of immigrants from Central America and Cuba. Use of the generic term *Hispanic* is problematic in that it glosses over cultural differences in subgroups and the specific needs each group might have. The term is used here with these limitations in mind.

Although early studies suggested that compared with Whites, Hispanics have lower rates of psychological distress, recent studies have suggested that the prevalence of psychological disorders among Hispanics may be at least a high as the general population, even when socioeconomic status is controlled for. With respect to symptoms of depression, several studies have found prevalence rates to be much higher than those found in the general population (81, 82). Moreover, Hispanic women have been found to have significantly higher levels of depressive symptomatology than do Hispanic men, even when age and education are controlled for (82). Roberts and Vernon (81) found a 27 percent lifetime prevalence rate for either major or minor depression, using the Schedule for Affective Disorders and Schizophrenia--Lifetime Version. In our study, the San Francisco Depression Prevention Research Project, we found a 38.1 percent lifetime prevalence rate of either major depression or dysthymia, on the basis of the Diagnostic Interview Schedule among Spanish-speaking primary care outpatients.

However, because of the dearth of epidemiological studies in communities with a high percentage of Hispanics, reliable estimates of prevalence of psychological disorders among Hispanics do not exist. The best estimates are forthcoming from the Los Angeles Epidemiologic Catchment Area study (83).

Most of the available literature points to underutilization of mental health services among Hispanics (84, 85). Underutilization has been attributed to characteristics of the mental health system (the lack of available services, in that existing clinics often discourage Hispanics from using services) or of the culture (stigma associated with receiving treatment, use of natural support systems to deal with emotional problems, use of traditional healers, or the low level of need for psychological services) (86, 87).

A few studies have reported that mental health service utilization among Hispanics is at least equal to that of other groups (88, 89). However, there continues to be a lack of available services to adequately meet the needs of the Hispanic population. Given the constant influx of immigrants from many Latin American countries, more bilingual Hispanic professionals are needed. These professionals need to have a firm knowledge of the social and political conditions leading to migration and the concomitant stressors faced by recent arrivals. But too few Hispanic professionals exist (90, 91). To help fill the gap, indigenous paraprofessionals are frequently used, especially in community mental health centers (92).

Given the lack of adequate services, there has been a growing recognition of the need for Hispanic preventive mental health services (93, 94) and research (91). Strategies for delivering these services also have been identified (95-97).

Prevention Services

It is known that community residents who seek treatment from Hispanic community mental health centers typically suffer from high levels of psychosocial stressors. In 1982, a one-time review conducted by one of us (R.A.) of all open charts of a San Francisco Bay Area community mental health center that specializes in serving Hispanics indicated that 40 percent of the center's client population suffered from psychosocial stressors rated severe, extreme, or catastrophic, according to Axis Four of the *DSM-III*.

The extent to which such high levels of psychosocial stressors exist in Hispanic communities in general is not known; however, Hispanic communities do have considerable stressors, given the high levels of unemployment/underemployment, problems with immigration status, and other factors.

Hispanic community mental health centers have attempted to address these problems by offering primary prevention services. Often these services have a particular cultural focus, such as building self-esteem in young children, or a problem focus, such as education on drug abuse or perinatal services. Usually these services are provided by paraprofessionals. The continued need for primary prevention services in community mental health has been documented (98).

Unfortunately, few of these centers have published descriptions or evaluations of their services. The available literature suggests that primary prevention services for children are often designed to prevent education failure (91) or behavior problems (99). Prevention services for adolescents and young adults include culture-specific prevention strategies for substance abuse among Hispanics (100) and child abuse prevention services for adolescent mothers (101). In the former example (100), a culture-specific primary prevention strategy is used to reduce acculturation stress and family conflicts, with the goal of preventing later drug abuse in children of these families. The services include family crisis intervention, bicultural effectiveness training, information on drug abuse, and family development training. No evaluative data of these centers are available, but the authors state that they expect this culture-specific intervention to be effective in reducing drug abuse in Hispanic families (100).

In Bolton et al.'s (101) study, 190 new adolescent mothers (38 percent were Hispanic, 31 percent were Black, 31 percent were White) who were judged to be at extreme risk for poor bonding and possible child maltreatment were identified by the staff at a county hospital. Home visits and a variety of social services were offered to those who were interested. Approximately 27 months after the program began, Child Protective Services records were reviewed. Eighteen families had been reported for possible child abuse or neglect, and the majority of these suspected cases were from the Anglo sample. These 18 families were compared with 172 families who did not report child maltreatment to identify high-risk factors for such behavior. The high-risk factors were related to poor parenting skills and low social supports. The authors suggested that preventive programs should be aimed at reducing these risk factors.

Mass media (television and radio) have been used in the Hispanic community to help the public learn to recognize mental health problems and identify service centers to treat these problems (97, 102). At other times, mass media have been used to address problems common to the Hispanic elderly (103). Although these programs were primarily outreach in nature, Muñoz (96) and Padilla et al. (91) suggested that this strategy could be used in primary prevention with Hispanics. In designing a prevention program for low-income populations, one may want to keep in mind efforts made in treatment outcome studies to bridge the class differences that typically exist between therapists and low-income clients. These studies have shown that bridging expectations tends to produce longer participation in treatment (104, 105). To increase the likelihood that prevention work will be effective with low-income and minority populations, it may be important to provide adequate education about the prevention goals and to make the intervention socially and culturally relevant.

Prevention Research

Johnson and Breckenridge (99) conducted a study designed to prevent behavior problems in young Chicano/Mexican children. Families were recruited through a neighborhood child development center: 128 children and their families were randomly assigned to either the intervention program or a control group. The intervention program offered a variety of supportive services, designed to meet the social and psychological needs of a recent immigrant population. The program encouraged the parental expression of affectionate behavior toward the children. Mothers were taught how to identify and respond to their children's developmental level and emotional states and how to manage their children using social learning and cognitive principles. The entire program consisted of approximately 500 hours of participation, spanning two years.

All families were followed over a five-year period, and evaluative data on the children's behavior were obtained by interviewing mothers. Control boys were judged to be significantly more destructive, overactive, and attention-seeking than intervention program boys. Boys in the intervention program condition and girls in both conditions presented few problems.

The authors noted weaknesses in the data, given that the ratings of the children's behavior were exclusively those of their mothers. Also, the study suffered a substantial dropout rate (48 percent for program families, 38 percent for control families). Only data on those families that completed the study in either condition were reported in this article.

Despite these weaknesses, the benefits of Johnson and Beckenridge's program continue to be shown. Preliminary analyses have indicated that the children in the intervention condition have higher IQs and significantly more work motivation than do controls. Moreover, the program may be benefitting other children in the family as well, which, the authors note, could increase the program's value and cost effectiveness.

A randomized mental health prevention study, still in progress, focuses on prevention with Hispanic women. The Hispanic Social Network Prevention Intervention Study (106) is a primary and secondary prevention study of depression that focuses on middle-aged, low-income Chicanas and immigrant Mexican women, who, because of various social and economic factors, are believed to be at high risk for depression. Prevention of the onset of depressive symptomatogy is being attempted by increasing personal coping resources and thereby improving self-concept (feelings of self-efficacy and mastery). Screening instruments were used to identify a target population of low-income Mexican women, aged 35-50, who have been living in the United States for at least two years and who were not experiencing high levels of depressive symptomatogy at the time of screening. The Center for Epidemiologic Studies Depression Scale (107), the Diagnostic Interview Schedule (19), and other screening instruments and baseline measures were used with respondents from a county-wide sample to select a stratified probability sample. With this procedure, 600 women are expected to be selected into the study and then will be randomly assigned to one of two prevention conditions or to a control group. Both prevention interventions begin with a three-month intensive phase, followed by nine months of periodic contact. Although participants are not paid for attending sessions, money is available in the budget to pay for babysitting costs.

One of the prevention modes focuses on the use of paraprofessionals as natural helpers (that is, *servidoras*) who, through building rapport in one-to-one relationships, help study participants cope with stressful life events. As needed, these servidoras link individuals to social resources. They also help participants develop, or restore, and expand their coping abilities by using techniques evolving from social learning theory.

The second prevention condition uses a peer group format, which they call *merienda educativa*. Based on the work done by Boulette (108) with low-income Chicanas and immigrant Mexicans, the design of this intervention is rooted in group dynamics. In addition to working with participants on an individual basis, the servidoras use the group to provide more formal instruction, as well as to encourage sharing of experiences, through which the coping repertoires and skills of group members may be increased. The women in the control group receive no intervention.

The Hispanic Social Network Prevention Intervention Study will identify population subgroups who are willing to participate in prevention trials. More important, it will help determine to what extent current psychological techniques may be useful in preventing the onset of depressive symptoms with low-income Hispanic women. High-risk factors of these women that may be reduced by the interventions may also be identified.

WHAT DO WE KNOW?

Our review of the literature indicates that there is a relatively large number of articles and chapters that propose primary prevention programs as logical and theoretically effective ways to protect minorities in the United States from psychological problems. Many of these articles argue that minority groups are more likely to use preventive services than treatment services. Advocates of this point of view hold that because preventive services can be provided in educational or other contexts, they involve little stigma for participants. It has also been recommended that preventive services be planned in consultation with the cultural groups to be served to increase the cultural appropriateness of the services and the community's acceptance of the program.

There are very few reports of true prevention programs in the literature. Many "preventive" programs are outreach programs which attempt to identify untreated cases and offer them treatment. These should be labeled secondary prevention programs, for they do not meet criteria for primary prevention. Many of these services appear to be temporary programs, usually the result of special projects led by an individual or group. Once the organizers move on or lose funding, the programs end.

There are even fewer primary prevention research studies. The vast majority of research studies focus on prevention of symptoms or promotion of mental health, rather than the prevention of specific disorders. Three randomized controlled prevention studies that focus on specific disorders are still in progress (18, 41, 106). None of the completed studies we found reported cost effectiveness data related to prevention of psychological problems.

RECOMMENDATIONS

Clarify the Definition of Primary Prevention

We found many articles in which the word *prevention* was used to refer to what were really outreach efforts to identify and treat cases. In order to make progress in the primary prevention area, it will be important to note that primary prevention efforts are aimed at "reducing the incidence of new cases of mental disorder and disability in a population" (109, p. 128). Cowen (110) adds an important definitional point: "Primary prevention activities are targeted impersonally to groups and communities; once individual distress is identified, intervention is other than primary" (p. 433). Primary prevention programs are provided to persons who belong to high-risk groups because of demographic characteristics, not because they have been found to have psychological dysfunctions. Thus, a program for single mothers under the poverty level would meet the criterion for primary prevention. A program that has screened single mothers, found those who meet *DSM-III* criteria for major depression, and offered them an intervention is not a primary prevention program. (However, it would most likely be an important and worthwhile early identification and treatment program.)

Specify the Cross-Cultural Groups Being Served

We believe that it is important both from a scientific and a socially conscious perspective to make sure that primary prevention projects and research studies involve representative samples of the community being served. This means that projects that take place in large urban areas will have to include members of at least some of the four groups we have discussed. It is important, then, to analyze results of the intervention by ethnic group.

In addition to the effectiveness of the intervention on those who receive it, part of the evaluation of services from a cross-cultural perspective includes evaluation of accessibility, availability, acceptability, appropriateness, and accountability (111). It has been pointed out that even "free access to comprehensive care does not itself assure fair shares of services or equity in benefits" (12, p. 89). The literature provides clear evidence that ethnic differences exist in the use of mental health services (112) and even in interpretation of and reaction to disaster warnings (113). If specific cultural groups underutilize services meant for the community, there is a duty in the part of the service providers to modify the services so that they are used (114). It is very important that individuals within service or research teams take their scientific and public health duties seriously and persist in reminding the team to not neglect specific groups (115). Providing culturally and linguistically appropriate services is expensive and takes a lot of energy and coordination; thus it is likely to be neglected if not strongly advocated by members of the team.

Use Standardized Measures

The controversy about the use of culturally appropriate measures is very complex and has no easy solution. In the San Francisco Depression Prevention Research Project we have chosen to use measures that have been widely used in United States community studies. We have used the forward-and-backward translation methods in order to be able to compare these measures across the many groups we work with. We realize that there may still be differences in the way the measures work, but we have decided to analyze this possibility empirically. In addition to using widely used scales, we also include in our batteries measures of biculturality to determine the effect of this variable on our core measures. Others may choose to use a common core of instruments across ethnic groups and add culturally specific measures when appropriate.

The construction and development of culturally specific measures is a long and expensive process. Even if such measures were developed, one is faced with the inherent lack of comparability with other studies and other populations. We believe it is more practical to use standard scales and empirically establish norms and determine their utility.

We strongly recommend the explicit collection of the symptoms that are used to determine current diagnostic criteria. Even if the diagnostic criteria change, the patterns of symptoms can be used to make comparisons across studies and, if appropriate, to determine whether new diagnostic criteria are met. For example, Kleinman (116), studying neurasthenia and depression in China, found that out of 100 patients diagnosed as having neurasthenia, 87 met *DSM-III* criteria for major depression and an additional 6 met criteria for dysthymia; cyclothymia; or manic-depression, depressed type. Without having to assume that we are merely calling the same disorder a different name, we can at least document that the symptoms being studied are the same and that they appear together as a syndrome with remarkable frequency. It is even possible that data bases composed of symptom information could be used to statistically derive syndromes that are universal and syndromes that are culturally specific.

Specify Your Prevention Strategy

At least three approaches have been specifically suggested for prevention intervention projects. We recommend that prevention teams explicitly state the framework that directs their efforts.

Health Promotion. Some advocates of prevention have rejected the prevention of specific disorders as an effective approach and advocate instead a health-directed (versus a disease-directed) model. For example, Rappaport (117) suggested that empowerment may be a better goal than prevention.

Reduction of Stressful Life Events or Their Negative Effects as a Nonspecific Prevention Strategy. The most forceful argument for the reduction of stressful life events or their negative effects as a nonspecific prevention strategy was made by Bloom (118). Briefly, he reminds us that because stress can increase the probability of a number of psychological and physical disorders, it makes more sense to focus on stress reduction interventions, which are likely to have a widespread effect on dysfunction of many kinds, rather than on prevention of specific diagnostic categories.

Disorder-Specific Interventions. This approach focuses on specific syndromes and attempts to intervene using information specific to the disorder. Note that the etiology of the disorder need not be known to prevent it, just as it need not be known to treat it effectively. As a matter of fact, effective preventive or treatment approaches may give us clues to its etiology.

In sum, we recommend that prevention teams focus on their preferred theoretical approach and allow the results to determine which is the best strategy. It is quite feasible to collect information on all three possibilities in the same study. For example, in the San Francisco Depression Prevention Research Project, we are collecting measures of positive change, diagnostic information on many *DSM-III* disorders, as well as information on depression itself.

Specify the Intervention to Be Used and Its Theoretical Basis

To best advance the prevention field, it is important that the theory behind the intervention be explicitly presented. The intervention itself also should be described well enough to be replicable. This is best done with the use of a detailed protocol.

Prevention interventions generally are focused on changing a set of mediating variables, such as the frequency of stressful events, the social support network, thinking patterns, behavioral patterns, income, and so on. It is important that these variables, which hypothetically produce the prevention effect, are measured before and after the intervention. If the theorized changes do not take place, the theory has not received an adequate test.

Whatever the prevention strategy chosen, it is the responsibility of the prevention team to ascertain whether they achieved their intended final outcome. Ideally, this final outcome includes information on the reduction of incidence of the identified disorder or specific symptoms. In addition, cost data regarding the intervention and possible cost offset would be most helpful to plan future work.

Merge Service Programs With Research Programs

Much of what we have learned from clinical research has come from hypotheses derived from clinical experience. It is important that we avoid the possibly wasteful option of building research programs based on armchair planning. We are more likely to make progress if researchers and prevention practitioners collaborate, bringing together front-line expertise with scientific rigor (119).

Emphasize Results Rather Than Process

We recommend that cross-culturally oriented prevention teams focus primarily on achieving prevention effects. We sense that such teams are sometimes immobilized by concerns of not being culturally sensitive or by not being able to specify how they are being "culturally appropriate." Perhaps we have reacted too strongly to the criticisms made of insensitive researchers and practitioners who barged (and, we are sure, still barge) into culturally different communities, causing resentment and counterproductive effects. What minority communities want is reduction in suffering. If we can produce this result and document it, making the benefits of the intervention clear and meaningful to the communities, we will have served them well. Cultural appropriateness can best be measured by whether the community makes use of the services, whether they rate the services as useful, whether the services produce preventive effects with the members of that community, and whether negative effects are minor or nonexistent.

Prevent Demoralization in Prevention Teams

Prevention of psychological and emotional suffering is a worthwhile human goal. It was worthwhile before public, professional, or government groups began to support it and will continue to be worthwhile even if organized support for it stops. Obviously, the more support we obtain, the faster progress will be made. But even if it takes much longer than we hope, whatever efforts we make now will eventually help to reach our ultimate goal of pushing back the boundaries of what is now considered unavoidable and inescapable.

When resources are withdrawn, when results are not as dazzling as we would like, we might find some inspiration in remembering that, in the long run, those who say it can't be done will be silenced by someone doing it.

REFERENCES

1. Marsella AJ: Cross-cultural studies of mental disorders, in Perspectives on Cross-Cultural Psychology. Edited by Marsella AJ, Tharp RG, Ciborowski TJ. New York, Academic Press, 1979

2. Higginbotham HN: Culture and mental health services, in Perspectives on Cross-Cultural Psychology. Edited by Marsella AJ, Tharp RG, Ciborowski TJ. New York, Academic Press, 1979

3. Draguns JG, Phillips L: Culture and Psychopathology: The Quest for a Relationship. Morristown, NJ, General Learning Press, 1972

4. Dohrenwend BP, Dohrenwend BS: The problem of validity in field studies of psychological disorder. J Abnorm Psychol 70:52-66, 1965

5. Marsella AJ: Depressive experience and disorder across cultures, in Handbook of Cross-Cultural Psychology: Volume 6. Psychopathology. Edited by Draguns J, Triandis H. Boston, Allyn and Bacon, 1980

6. Dohrenwend BP, Dohrenwend BS: Social and cultural influences on psychopathology. Ann Rev Psychol 25:417-452, 1974

7. Dohrenwend BP, Dohrenwend BS: Socioenvironmental factors, stress, and psychopathology. Am J Community Psychol 9:128-159, 1981

8. Boyd JH, Weissman MM: Epidemiology, in Handbook of Affective Disorders. Edited by Paykel ES. New York, Guilford, 1982

9. Brown GW, Harris T: Social Origins of Depression. New York, Free Press, 1978

10. U.S. Department of Health, Education, and Welfare: Healthy People: The Surgeon General's Report on Health Promotion and Disease Prevention (Publication No. PHS 79-55071). Washington, DC, U.S. Government Printing Office, 1979

11. Hamburg DA, Elliott GR, Parron DL (Editors): Health and Behavior: Frontiers of Research in the Biobehavioral Sciences. Washington, DC, National Academy Press, 1982

12. Morris JN: Social inequalities undiminished. Lancet 1:87-90, 1979

13. Hayes-Bautista D: Raza demographics and social policy, in Issues in Latino Health. Presented at a meeting of the Bay Area Latino Health Sciences Faculty Network, Berkeley, CA, March 1983

14. Talbott JA: Social Issues and Decisions That Will Effect Change in the Practice of Psychiatry. Paper presented at the annual meeting of the American Psychiatric Association, Washington, DC, May 1985

15. National Institute of Mental Health: Preventing the Harmful Consequences of Severe and Persistent Loneliness (Publication No. ADM 84-1312). Edited by Peplau LA, Goldston SE.

Washington, DC, U.S. Government Printing Office, 1984
16. U.S. Bureau of the Census: Statistical Abstract of the United States: 1984 (104th Edition). Washington, DC, 1983
17. National Institute of Mental Health: Primary Prevention in Mental Health: An Annotated Bibliography (Publication No. ADM 85-1405). Edited by Buckner JC, Trickett EJ, Corse SJ. Washington, DC, U.S. Government Printing Office, 1985
18. Muñoz RF, Ying YW, Armas R, et al: The San Francisco Depression Prevention Research Project: a randomized trial with medical outpatients, in Depression Prevention: Research Directions. Edited by Muñoz RF. New York, Hemisphere, in press
19. Robins LN, Helzer JE, Croughan J, et al: National Institute of Mental Health Diagnostic Interview Schedule: its history, characteristics, and validity. Arch Gen Psychiatry 38:381-389, 1981
20. Robins LN, Helzer JE, Ratcliff KS, et al: Validity of the Diagnostic Interview Schedule, Version 2: DSM-III diagnosis. Psychol Med 12:855-870, 1982
21. American Psychiatric Association: Diagnostic and Statistical Manual of Mental Disorders (Third Edition). Washington, DC, American Psychiatric Association, 1980
22. Lewinsohn PM, Muñoz RF, Youngren MA, et al: Control Your Depression (Revised Edition). New York, Prentice-Hall, 1986
23. Manson SM, Tatum E, Dinges NG: Prevention research among American Indian and Alaska Native communities: charting future courses for theory and practice in mental health, in New Directions in Prevention Among American Indian and Alaska Native Communities. Edited by Manson SM. Portland, OR, Oregon Health Sciences University, 1982
24. Shore JH, Kinzie JD, Hampson JL: Psychiatric epidemiology of an Indian village. Psychiatry 36:70-81, 1973
25. Roy C, Chaudhuri A, Irvine D: The prevalence of mental disorders among Saskatchewan Indians. Journal of Cross-Cultural Psychology 1:383-392, 1970
26. Sampath BM: Prevalence of psychiatric disorders in a southern Baffin Island Eskimo settlement. Can Psychiatric Assoc J 19:303-367, 1974
27. Ostendorf D, Hammerschlag CA: An Indian-controlled mental health program. Hosp Community Psychiatry 28:682-685, 1977
28. Beiser M, Attneave CL: Mental disorders among American Indian children: rates and risk periods for entering treatment. Am J Psychiatry 139:193-198, 1982
29. Manson SM, Trimble JE: Mental health services to American

Indian and Alaska Native communities: past efforts, future inquiry, in Reaching the Underserved: Mental Health Needs of Neglected Populations. Edited by Snowden LR. Beverly Hills, CA, Sage, 1982

30. Trimble JE: Value differentials and their importance in counseling American Indians, in Counseling Across Cultures (Second Edition). Edited by Draguns J, Lonner W, Trimble J. Honolulu, University Press of Hawaii, 1981
31. Dinges N, Trimble J, Manson S, et al: The social ecology of counseling and psychotherapy with American Indians and Alaska Natives, in Cross-Cultural Counseling and Psychotherapy: Foundations, Evaluation, Cultural Considerations. Edited by Marsella A, Pederson P. Elmsford, NJ, Pergamon Press, 1981
32. Trimble JE: American Indian mental health and the role of training for prevention, in New Directions in Prevention Among American Indian and Alaska Native Communities. Edited by Manson SM. Portland, OR, Oregon Health Sciences University, 1982
33. Red Horse J: American Indian community mental health: a primary prevention strategy, in New Directions in Prevention Among American Indian and Alaska Native Communities. Edited by Manson SM. Portland, OR, Oregon Health Sciences University, 1982
34. Shore JH, Keepers G: Examples of evaluation research in delivering preventive mental health services to Indian youth, in New Directions in Prevention Among American Indian and Alaska Native Communities. Edited by Manson SM. Portland, OR, Oregon Health Sciences University, 1982
35. Shore JH, Nicholls WM: Indian children and tribal group homes: new interpretations of the whipper man. Am J Psychiatry 132:454-456, 1975
36. Carpenter RA, Lyons CA, Miller WR: Peer-managed self-control program for prevention of alcohol abuse in American Indian high school students: a pilot evaluation study. Int J Addict 20:299-310, 1985
37. Haven GA, Imotichey PJ: Mental health services for American Indians: the USET program. White Cloud Journal 1:3-5, 1979
38. Kleinfeld J: Getting it together at adolescence: case studies of positive socializing environments for Eskimo youth, in New Directions in Prevention Among American Indian and Alaska Native Communities. Edited by Manson SM. Portland, OR, Oregon Health Sciences University, 1982
39. Mohatt G, Blue AW: Primary prevention as it relates to tradi-

tionality and empirical measures of social deviance, in New Directions in Prevention Among American Indian and Alaska Native Communities. Edited by Manson SM. Portland, OR, Oregon Health Sciences University, 1982

40. Dinges N: Mental health promotion with Navajo families, in New Directions in Prevention Among American Indian and Alaska Native Communities. Edited by Manson SM. Portland, OR, Oregon Health Sciences University, 1982

41. Manson SM: Depression Among Physically Ill Older American Indians: Planning the Design, Implementation and Evaluation of a Preventive Intervention. Paper presented at the Conference Medical Anthropology: Implementations for Stress Prevention Among Different Populations. Portland, OR, Oregon Health Sciences University, May 1984

42. Mamak A: American Indian Samoan Preventive Intervention Project. Paper presented at the Conference on Medical Anthropology: Implementations for Stress Prevention Among Different Populations. Portland, OR, Oregon Health Sciences University, May 1984

43. U.S. Department of Health and Human Services: Report to Congress: Refugee Resettlement Program. Washington, DC, U.S. Government Printing Office, 1984

44. Hatanaka HD, Watanabe BY, Ono S: The utilization of mental health services in the Los Angeles area, in Service Delivery in Pan Asian Communities. Edited by Ishikawa WH, Archer NH. San Diego, Pacific Asian Coalition, 1975

45. Sue S, McKinney H: Asian Americans in community health care systems. Am J Orthopsychiatry 45:111-118, 1975

46. Sue S, Morishima JK: The Mental Health of Asian Americans. San Francisco, CA, Jossey-Bass, 1982

47. Tung TM: Psychiatric care for Southeast Asians: how different is different? in Southeast Asian Mental Health: Treatment, Prevention, Services, Training, and Research (Publication No. ADM 85-1399). Edited by Owan TC. Rockville, MD, National Institute of Mental Health, 1985

48. Lin KM, Inui TS, Kleinman AM, et al: Sociocultural determinants of the help-seeking behavior of patients with mental illness. J Nerv Ment Dis 170:78-85, 1982

49. Sue S, Sue DW: MMPI comparisons between Asian-American and non-Asian students utilizing a student health psychiatric clinic. Journal of Counseling Psychology 21:423-427, 1974

50. Cheung FM, Lau BWK, Waldmann E: Somatization among Chinese depressives in general practice. Int J Psychiatry Medicine 10:361-374, 1981

51. Plaut T: Primary prevention in the '80s, in Community Sup-

port Systems and Mental Health. Edited by Biegal DE, Naparsek AJ. New York, Springer, 1982

52. Owan TC (Editor): Southeast Asian Mental Health: Treatment, Prevention, Services, Training, and Research (Publication No. ADM 85-1399). Rockville, MD, National Institute of Mental Health, 1985

53. Yee T, Lee R: Based on cultural strengths: a school primary prevention program for Asian-American youth. Community Ment Health J 13:239-248, 1977

54. Carlin JE, Sokoloff BZ: Mental health treatment issues for Southeast Asian refugee children, in Southeast Asian Mental Health: Treatment, Prevention, Services, Training, and Research (Publication No. ADM 85-1399). Edited by Owan TC. Rockville, MD, National Institute of Mental Health, 1985

55. Khoa LX, Bui DD: Southeast Asian mutual assistance association: an approach for community development, in Southeast Asian Mental Health: Treatment, Prevention, Services, Training, and Research (Publication No. ADM 85-1399). Edited by Owan TC. Rockville, MD, National Institute of Mental Health, 1985

56. Waltis C, Dolan BB: Day care centers for the old. Time, January 18, 1982, p. 60

57. Zawadski R, Shen J, Yordi C, et al: On Lok: A Research and Development Project. San Francisco, On Lok Senior Health Services, 1985

58. Adebimpe VR: Overview: white norms and psychiatric diagnosis of black patients. Am J Psychiatry 137:679-682, 1980

59. Flaherty JA, Meagher R: Measuring racial bias in inpatient treatment. Am J Psychiatry 137:679-682, 1980

60. Sue S: Community mental health services to minority groups: some optimism, some pessimism. Am Psychol 32:616-624, 1977

61. Mollica RF, Redlich F: Equity and changing patient characteristics--1950 to 1975. Arch Gen Psychiatry 37:1257-1263, 1980

62. Sue S, Allen D, McKinney H, et al: Delivery of community mental health services to black and white clients. J Consult Clin Psychol 42:794-801, 1974

63. Eaton W, Kessler L: Rates of symptoms of depression in a national sample. Am J Epidemiol 114:528-538, 1981

64. Roberts R, Stevenson J, Breslow L: Symptoms of depression among blacks and whites in an urban community. J Nerv Ment Dis 169:774-779, 1981

65. Neighbors HW: The distribution of psychiatric morbidity in black Americans: a review and suggestions for research. Com-

munity Ment Health J 20:169-181, 1984

66. Robins LN, Helzer JE, Weissman MM, et al: Lifetime prevalence of specific psychiatric disorders in three sites. Arch Gen Psychiatry 41:949-958, 1984

67. Glasscote RM, Kohn E, Beigel A, et al: Preventing Mental Illness: Efforts and Attitudes. Washington, DC, Joint Information Service of the American Psychiatric Association and the Mental Health Association, 1980

68. Paster VS: Organizing primary prevention programs with disadvantaged community groups, in Primary Prevention: An Idea Whose Time Has Come (Publication No. ADM 80-447). Edited by Klein DC, Goldston SE. Rockville, MD, National Institute of Mental Health, 1985

69. Heber FR, Garber H, Harrington S, et al: Rehabilitation of Families at Risk for Mental Retardation. Madison, University of Wisconsin, 1972

70. Heber FR: Sociocultural mental retardation: a longitudinal study, in Primary Prevention of Psychopathology: Volume 2. Environmental Influences. Edited by Forgays DG. Hanover, NH, University Press of New England, 1978

71. Shure MB: Training children to solve interpersonal problems: a preventive mental health program, in Social and Psychological Research in Community Settings. Edited by Muñoz RF, Snowden LR, Kelly JG. San Francisco, Jossey-Bass, 1979

72. Shure MB, Spivack G: Interpersonal problem solving thinking and adjustment in the mother-child dyad, in Social Competence in Children. Edited by Kent MW, Rolf JE. Hanover, NH, University Press of New England, 1979

73. Shure MB, Spivack G: Interpersonal problem solving in young children: a cognitive approach to prevention. Am J Community Psychol 10:341-356, 1982

74. Goldston SE: A national perspective, in Primary Prevention of Psychopathology: Volume 2: Environmental Influences. Edited by Forgays DG. Hanover, NH, University Press of New England, 1978

75. Felner RD, Ginter M, Primavera J: Primary prevention during school transitions: social support and environmental structure. Am J Community Psychol 10:277-290, 1982

76. Bry BH: Reducing the incidence of adolescent problems through preventive intervention: one- and five-year follow-up. Am J Community Psychol 10:265-276, 1982

77. Bry BH, George FE: Evaluating and improving prevention programs: a strategy for drug abuse. Evaluation and Program Planning 2:127-136, 1979

78. Bry BH, George FE: The preventive effects of early interven-

tion on the attendance and grades of urban adolescents. Professional Psychology 11:252-260, 1980

79. Gatz M, Barbarin OA, Tyler FB, et al: Enhancement of individual and community competence: the older adult as community worker. Am J Community Psychol 10:291-304, 1982

80. Muñoz RF: The Spanish-speaking consumer and the community mental health center, in Minority Mental Health. Edited by Jones EE, Korchin SJ. New York, Praeger, 1982

81. Roberts RE, Vernon SW: Minority status and psychological distress reexamined: the case of Mexican Americans. Research in Community and Mental Health 4:131-164, 1984

82. Vernon SW, Roberts RE: Use of SADS-RDC in a tri-ethnic community survey. Arch Gen Psychiatry 39:47-52, 1982

83. Hough R, Karno M, Burnham MA, et al: The Los Angeles Epidemiologic Catchment Area Research Program and the epidemiology of psychiatric disorders among Mexican Americans. J Operational Psychiatry 14:43-51, 1983

84. Keefe SE, Padilla AM, Carlos ML: Emotional Support Systems in Two Cultures: a Comparison of Mexican Americans and Anglo Americans (Occasional Paper No. 7). Los Angeles, Spanish-Speaking Mental Health Research Center, 1978

85. Padilla AM, Ruiz RA: Latino Mental Health: a Review of the Literature (Publication No. ADM 76-113). Washington, DC, U.S. Government Printing Office, 1973

86. Barrera M Jr: Raza populations, in Reaching the Underserved: Mental Health Needs of Neglected Populations. Edited by Snowden LR. Beverly Hills, CA, Sage, 1982

87. Keefe SE, Casas JM: Mexican Americans and mental health: a selected review and recommendations for mental health service delivery. Am J Community Psychol 8:303-326, 1980

88. Trevino FM, Bruhn JG: Incidence of mental illness in a Mexican American community. Psychiatric Annals 7:33-51, 1977

89. Wignall CM, Koppin LL: Mexican American image of state mental hospital facilities. Community Ment Health J 3:137-148, 1967

90. Trevino AL, Lopez S: Professional Hispanic personnel: an annotated bibliography, in Hispanic Mental Health Professionals (Monograph No. 5). Edited by Olmedo EL, Lopez S. Los Angeles, Spanish-Speaking Mental Health Research Center, 1977

91. Padilla AM, Lindholm KJ: Hispanic behavioral science research: recommendations for future research. Hispanic Journal of Behavioral Sciences 6:13-32, 1984

92. Flores-Ortiz YG: Indigenous paraprofessionals in mental

health: an analysis and critique, in Reaching the Underserved:
Mental Health Needs of Neglected Populations. Edited by
Snowden LR. Beverly Hills, CA, Sage, 1982

93. Keefe SE, Casas JM: Family and mental health among
Mexican Americans: some considerations for mental health
services, in Family and Mental Health in the Mexican American Community (Monograph No. 7). Edited by Casas JM,
Keefe SE. Los Angeles, Spanish-speaking Mental Health Research Center, 1978

94. Levine ES, Padilla AM: Crossing Cultures in Therapy:
Pluralistic Counseling for the Hispanic. Monterey,
Brooks/Cole, 1980

95. Cohen RE: Principles of preventive mental health programs
for ethnic minority populations: the acculturation of Puerto
Ricans to the United States. Am J Psychiatry 128:1529-1533,
1972

96. Munoz RF: A strategy for the prevention of psychological
problems in Latinos: emphasizing accessibility and effectiveness, in Hispanic Natural Support Systems. Edited by Valle R,
Vega W. Sacramento, California Department of Mental Health,
1980

97. Romero JT: Hispanic support systems: health-mental health
promotion strategies, in Hispanic Natural Support Systems.
Edited by Valle R, Vega W. Sacramento, California Department of Mental Health, 1980

98. President's Commission on Mental Health: Report to the
President. Washington, DC, U.S. Department of Health and
Human Services, 1978

99. Johnson DL, Breckenridge JN: The Houston parent-child
development center and the primary prevention of behavior
problems in young children. Am J Community Psychol
10:305-316, 1982

100. Santisteban D, Szapocznik J: Substance abuse disorders among
Hispanics: a focus on prevention, in Mental Health, Drug, and
Alcohol Abuse: An Hispanic Assessment of Present and Fu-
ture Challenges. Edited by Szapocznik J. Washington, DC,
National Coalition of Hispanic Mental Health and Human
Services Organization, 1979

101. Bolton FG Jr, Charlton JR, Gai DS, et al: Preventive screening of adolescent mothers and infants: critical variables in
assessing risk for child maltreatment. J Primary Prevention
5:169-187, 1985

102. Boulette TR: Problemas familiares: television programs in
Spanish for mental health education. Hosp Community Psychiatry 25:2-82, 1974

103. Szapocznik J, Lasaga J, Perry P, et al: Outreach in the delivery of mental health services to Hispanic elders. Hispanic Journal of Behavioral Sciences 1:21-40, 1979
104. Jacobs SC, Charles E, Jacobs T, et al: Preparation for treatment of the disadvantaged patient: effects on disposition and outcome. Am J Orthopsychiatry 42:666-674, 1972
105. Acosta FX, Yamamoto J, Evans LA: Effective Psychotherapy for Low-Income and Minority Patients. New York, Plenum Press, 1982
106. Vega W, Valle R, Kolody B, et al: The Hispanic social network prevention intervention study: a community-based randomized trial, in Depression Prevention: Research Directions. Edited by Muñoz RF. New York, Hemisphere Press, in press
107. Radloff LS: The CES-D scale: A self-report depression scale for research in the general population. Applied Psychological Measurement 1:385-401, 1977
108. Boulette TR: Priority issues for mental health promotion among low-income Chicanos/Mexicanos, in Hispanic Natural Support Systems. Edited by Valle R, Vega W. Sacramento, California Department of Mental Health, 1980
109. Caplan G, Grunebaum H: Perspectives on primary prevention: a review, in The Critical Issues of Community Mental Health. Edited by Gottesfeld H. New York, Behavioral Publications, 1972
110. Cowen EL: Social and community interventions. Annual Review of Psychology 24:423-472, 1973
111. Owan TC: Neighborhood based mental health: an approach to overcome inequities in mental health services delivery to social and ethnic minorities, in Community Support Systems and Mental Health: Practice, Policy, and Research. Edited by Biegel DE, Naparstek AJ. New York, Springer, 1980
112. Barrera M Jr: Mexican-American mental health service utilization: a critical examination of some proposed variables. Community Ment Health J 14:35-45, 1978
113. Perry RW, Lindell MK, Greene MR: Crisis communications: ethnic differentials in interpreting and acting on disaster warnings. Social Behavior and Personality 10:97-104, 1982
114. Muñoz RF: Commentary. (On Pope S, Winslade WJ: "Unequal access to mental health services: the challenge to professional integrity"). Business and Professional Ethics Journal, in press
115. Maccoby N, Alexander J: Reducing heart disease risk using the mass media: comparing the effects on three communities, in Social and Psychological Research in Community Settings. Edited by Muñoz RF, Snowden LR, Kelly JG. San Francisco,

Jossey-Bass, 1979
116. Kleinman AM: Neurasthenia and depression: a study of somatization and culture in China. Cult Med Psychiatry 6:117-190, 1982
117. Rappaport J: In praise of paradox: a social policy of empowerment over prevention. Am J Community Psychol 9:1-25, 1981
118. Bloom BL: Stressful Life Event Theory and Research: Implications for Primary Prevention (Publication No. ADM 85-1385). Washington, DC, U.S. Government Printing Office, 1985
119. Muñoz RF: Primary prevention: should we support both practice and research? Journal of Primary Prevention 5:284-292, 1985

3

Primary Prevention
and Child Development

Leon Eisenberg, M.D.

3

Primary Prevention
and Child Development

Before considering how to undertake primary prevention of psychiatric disorders in children, it is important to consider why prevention is worthwhile. The one compelling reason is to improve health. However, government policy statements embrace prevention for a different reason: as a way to control costs. In its *Forward Plan for Health,* the U.S. Department of Health, Education, and Welfare heralded its new emphasis on prevention, stating, "The primary focus of our program is a major attack on cost escalation as the factor now driving national health policy" (1, p. 2). The same purpose has been voiced by Canada (2), the United Kingdom (3), and the Organization for Economic Cooperation and Development (4).

The goal of controlling costs of health care is surely understandable. But will prevention control costs? And is cost saving an appropriate standard for evaluating preventive medicine?

The answers to these questions may seem self-evident if one considers that immunization against poliomyelitis (5), pertussis, measles, and rubella (6) costs far less than treatment of those diseases and their sequelae. On the other hand, vaccinating the elderly against influenza costs an additional $2,000 per year of life gained because of medical costs in the added years (7). Free erythrocyte protoporphyrin screening for presymptomatic lead poisoning in three-year-olds saves money only when the prevalence of lead poisoning is seven percent or higher (8). Acceptance of cost effectiveness as the appropriate standard for evaluating preventive medicine implies that the health benefits of influenza vaccination to the elderly and screening for presymptomatic lead poisoning to children in a less-than-seven-percent-prevalence environment should be foregone (9).

Increases in costs are inevitable not only despite prevention but to some extent because of it. For example, preventing premature death among adults increases the number of individuals in the population who survive to age 65 and older, the time of life when infirmities increase the need for care (10). Effective prevention will continue to cause some degree of cost increase until a research breakthrough facilitates the ability to avert the chronic diseases that accumulate with age (11). This does not diminish the case for prevention when it is weighed on a scale of human values; it does make evident the danger of basing its justification on economic grounds.

What measures of demonstrated health benefits effectiveness are available now to prevent psychiatric disorders in children? There are means of protecting the integrity of the central nervous system and means of enhancing psychosocial development. This division is convenient, but one should keep in mind that it oversimplifies reality (12). Brain damage not only increases the risk for psychopathology and subnormality but also renders the individual more vulnerable to environmental adversities (13). Moderate insults to the brain, which have no detectable aftermath in a favorable environment, add to the dysfunctions exhibited by children reared in a stressful one.

PROTECTING THE INTEGRITY
OF THE CENTRAL NERVOUS SYSTEM

Prenatal Care

Low birth weight is associated with higher rates of neonatal mortality and of neuropsychiatric morbidity among survivors (14). The single most powerful predictor of the probability of low birth weight is the socioeconomic class of the mother (15). This reflects the combined effects of the mother's inadequate nutrition (both before and during pregnancy), delay in obtaining obstetrical care, poor health habits, and increased life stress. Yet, despite the persistence of other unfavorable environmental features, access to proper obstetrical care (16) and supplemental nutrition during pregnancy (17) have been shown to reduce the proportion of low birth weight infants born to mothers at risk.

Smoking during pregnancy increases the chances of premature birth, with its attendant risks (18). Although physician-initiated efforts to discourage smoking in the general population have met with limited success, they have been more successful with pregnant women (19).

Excess alcohol intake during pregnancy can result in fetal alcohol syndrome (20) as well as fetal wastage, low birth weight, and congenital anomalies short of the full syndrome (21). Pregnant women who smoke and abuse alcohol double these risks. Health education can help change maternal behavior during pregnancy. During a media campaign to prevent fetal alcohol syndrome in Seattle, the number of women reporting any alcohol use at the time of the first prenatal visit dropped from 81 to 42 percent (22).

Maternal rubella during the first trimester of pregnancy places the fetus at severe risk for the congenital rubella syndrome, the stigmata of which include severe mental retardation and autism. Once the mother has been infected, therapeutic abortion is the only option. Rubella vaccination for preschool children has led to a sharp drop in the incidence of childhood rubella and a change in the age distribution of cases. By 1980, a reduction in the incidence of rubella in 15- to 19-year-olds became evident as the cohort vaccinated 10 years earlier reached late adolescence (23).

Amniocentesis between the 15th and 16th week of pregnancy permits the intrauterine diagnosis of a number of major central nervous system disorders and makes selective abortion an option. About one-third of cases of severe mental subnormality result from trisomy 21, the risk for which is about 1 in 1,000 for all births but rises to about 1 in 300 among mothers aged 35 to 39 and to 1 in 50 among mothers age 40 and older. Although a decrease in the percentage of births to women age 35 and older accounted for an estimated 26 percent decrease in Down's syndrome incidence between 1960 and 1975 (24), fertility rates in this group are projected to increase 37 percent in the 1980s. This is for two reasons: the greater number of women in this age cohort as the baby boom generation matures (25) and deferred pregnancies (26). Unless we provide adequate prenatal diagnostic facilities, an increase in the number of infants born with Down's syndrome will result.

Screening of pregnant women for serum alpha-fetoprotein followed by amniocentesis and ultrasonography among those with levels more than 2.5 times the median alpha-fetoprotein value for the population permits the identification of fetuses with neural tube defects. Selective abortion prevents the multiple severe handicaps (paralysis, incontinence, and mental subnormality) found in the majority of such infants and removes a source of great distress for families (27), including a high divorce rate (28).

Neonatal Screening

Screening tests for phenylketonuria and congenital hypothyroidism permit their detection in time to institute measures that can prevent mental subnormality (29, 30). Screening must be associated with a sophisticated biochemical diagnostic assessment of each case. Despite excellent technical performance, a screening program can fail because of lack of funds and facilities, public education, case retrieval, continuing medical care, and counseling (31).

Success in treating children with phenylketonuria has given rise to a second-order problem: the hazard to infants born to successfully treated women. Maternal hyperphenylalaninemia during pregnancy leads to microcephaly and cardiac malformations. Risk can be reduced by putting women with this disorder on a low-phenylalanine diet before they attempt to become pregnant. If introduced after pregnancy occurs, the diet brings little benefit because of damage done during the first six weeks of fetal development (32).

Preventing Environmental Hazards to the Brain

Accidents and poisonings are the leading causes of childhood and adolescent mortality and morbidity in the United States. Brain damage from head trauma can be minimized by vehicle accident control measures including speed limits; car safety restraints; automatically released air bags; better highway design; crash helmets for skateboard, bicycle, and motorcycle users; and appropriate traffic regulation. How little we have done is illustrated by the fact that accidents accounted for more than 24 percent of the total years of potential life lost in the United States in 1984 (33). Childhood poisonings have been markedly reduced since the introduction of safety caps on medication bottles and on common household disinfectants and other hazardous chemicals (34). Blood lead levels that result in relatively minor symptoms in adults can impair intellectual performance in children (35). Stricter environmental protection standards have led to lower blood lead levels among American children (36), but the smelting and oil industries continue to oppose environmental protection efforts.

Immunization in Childhood

Active immunization against diphtheria, pertussis, tetanus, poliomyelitis, measles, mumps, and rubella minimizes the neuropsychiatric sequelae of these diseases. For example, as the incidence of measles has declined sharply, so has the occurrence of subacute sclerosing panencephalitis (23). To this list, we must now take steps to add immunization against Hemophilus influenzae type b (37). It is intolerable, in view of the enormous benefit to children, that we have not yet attained complete immunization of all children in the population.

ENHANCING PSYCHOSOCIAL DEVELOPMENT

Vaccination has become the paradigm for prevention: It is an inexpensive measure that need be applied only once or at most a few times to yield permanent immunity. Unfortunately, no such model exists for the prevention of psychosocial disorders. There is not now in existence, nor will there ever be, a short-term psychiatric intervention that confers permanent immunity to later challenge. Why should this be so?

Development is an epigenetic process. Successful negotiation of one stage of development makes successful passage through the next more likely, but it does not ensure it. The organism faces new adaptive challenges at each new level of behavioral organization and requires additional inputs. Food is as specific a preventive for malnutrition as vaccination is for smallpox. But seeing that a child is well fed in the first year of life confers no protection against malnutrition in the next year. The effects of undernutrition differ with age but there is no age at which food is not necessary. Similarly, the psychosocial needs of infant, child and adolescent differ during development, but those needs must be met throughout the life span (12).

Three psychosocial measures have been proposed for the reduction of psychiatric disorders in childhood and adolescence: family planning, preschool intervention programs, and good schooling.

Family Planning

Children and their mothers show increased rates of psychiatric morbidity when mothers have too many children (38), when children are born to mothers who are too young (39-41), and when children are born unwanted (42, 43). Currently available methods of contraception and abortion have sharply reduced this burden. Reproductive mortality in the United States has fallen 73 percent over the past 20 years (44). The increase in legal abortions since 1967 has been the biggest factor in the reduction of neonatal mortality (45). Although first-trimester abortion yields less than one-tenth the mortality associated with pregnancy continuation among teenagers (46), although it does not impair subsequent pregnancy outcomes (47, 48), and although it results in improved psychosocial adjustment among women with unwanted pregnancies (49), abortion is no substitute for contraception.

Among industrialized countries, the United States has the highest pregnancy rate and the highest birth rate among women under 20, despite having the highest abortion rate. This is because it also has the lowest rate of contraceptive use (50). Yet few states mandate family life education in the public schools. Child psychiatrists must take the lead in advocating effective methods to educate adolescents for responsible sexuality.

Preschool Intervention Programs

Children from families of low socioeconomic status exhibit a cumulative disadvantage with increasing age on tests of academic achievement (51). Family background is the crucial variable in predicting scholastic outcome. This developmental attrition is by far the major problem in child psychiatry. The unhappy history of school failure is embedded in a matrix of conduct disorders, unsatisfactory work patterns, and antisocial behavior. The repetition of this sequence through cycles of disadvantage (52) burdens both families and communities. Can bad outcomes among families at risk be minimized?

The most recent findings from the follow-up of children enrolled in preschool enrichment programs provide convincing evidence that we can minimize bad outcomes among families at risk (53). The Ypsilanti study (54) demonstrated higher rates for high school graduation and continuing education, better employment records, less use of welfare, less incidence of adolescent pregnancy, and fewer violations of law among experimentals than among controls at age 19, 15 years after the intervention. The findings of a just-completed New York City study (55) are remarkably similar: better rates for employment, high school graduation, and college or vocational training, as well as more positive self-concepts at ages 19 to 21 among experimentals than among neighborhood controls. The challenge for social policy is to ensure that high-quality early education is available to all disadvantaged children.

Good Schooling

Extending preschool programs that involve families as active participants is only the first step. We must build on the gains they make possible by improving the quality of schooling. Rutter et al. (56) found that schools make a significant difference in behavioral as well as academic outcomes. Their study tracked cohorts of students whose characteristics were measured at time of entering secondary schools. Outcomes were significantly correlated with independent measures of school quality. Although social class differences persisted, good schools enhanced attainments among both middle- and lower class children.

IMPLICATIONS FOR PSYCHIATRIC POLICY

Scientific understanding of the basic processes of psychosocial development admittedly remains limited. If any area warrants a sustained financial commitment to fundamental research, surely the ecology of child development is that area. Yet what is to be done in the meantime, a meantime that is likely to be a long time? Today it is argued by some that social welfare programs must be deferred at a time of budget constraints. This argument accepts without challenge the present Federal budget's extensive expenditures for nuclear weapons and research and development of outer-space defense systems, which jeopardize rather than defend our national security (57, 58). Pentagon appropriations over the past four years totaled one *trillion*, seven billion, nine hundred million dollars (59). The choice is clear: Decisions made in favor of armaments reduce the options for health care (60). Evidence is already at hand in the recently reported increases in infant mortality in a number of states in parallel with Federal program cutbacks and consequent economic privation (61).

Children are exquisitely sensitive to time. Developmental needs must be met or development will falter. Providing the best care we know how to give does not guarantee us a trouble-free future; nothing can guarantee that. All we can expect is that better beginnings improve the odds for happier endings. Mental health professionals must become forceful advocates for the effectiveness of prevention of psychiatric disorders via protection of the integrity of the brain and enhancement of psychosocial development.

REFERENCES

1. U.S. Department of Health, Education and Welfare: A Forward Plan for Health: Fiscal Year 1978-82 (Publication No. OS76-50046). Washington, DC, U.S. Government Printing Office, 1976
2. Lalonde M: A New Perspective on the Health of Canadians. Ottawa, Canadian Government Printing Office, 1974
3. Prevention and Health: Everybody's Business. Prepared jointly by the health departments of Britain and Northern Ireland. London, HM Stationary Office, 1976

4. Organization for Economic Cooperation and Development: Public Expenditure on Health (Studies in Resource Allocation, No. 5). Paris, Organization for Economic Cooperation and Development, 1977

5. Fudenberg HH: Fiscal returns of biomedical research. J Invest Dermatol 61:321-329, 1973

6. Willens JS, Sanders CR: Cost-effectiveness and cost-benefit analyses of vaccines. J Infect Dis 144:486-493, 1981

7. U.S. Congress Office of Technology Assessment: Cost effectiveness of influenza vaccination. Washington, DC, U.S. Government Printing Office, 1981

8. Berwick DM, Komaroff AL: Cost-effectiveness of lead screening. N Engl J Med 306:1392-1398, 1982

9. Avorn J: Benefit and cost analysis in geriatric care: turning age discrimination into health policy. N Engl J Med 31:1294-1301, 1984

10. Gori GB, Richter BJ: Macroeconomics of disease prevention in the United States. Science 200:1124-1130, 1978

11. Rice DP, Estes CL: Health of the elderly: policy issues and challenges. Health Affairs 3:26-49, 1984

12. Eisenberg L: Development as a unifying concept. Br J Psychiatry 131:225-237, 1977

13. Rutter M: Psychological sequelae of brain damage in childhood. Am J Psychiatry 138:1533-1544, 1981

14. McCormick MC: The contribution of low birth weight to infant mortality and childhood morbidity. N Engl J Med 312:82-90, 1985

15. Rosen M: The biological vulnerability of the low birth weight infant, in Infants at Risk for Developmental Dysfunction. Washington, DC, National Academy of Sciences, Institute of Medicine, 1982

16. Goldman F, Grossman M: The Impact of Public Health Policy: The Case of Community Health Centers. Cambridge, MA, National Bureau of Economic Research, 1982

17. Kotelchuck M, Schwartz J, Anderka M, et al: WIC participation and pregnancy outcomes: Massachusetts statewide evaluation project. Am J Public Health 74:1086-1092, 1984

18. Koop E: The Health Consequences of Smoking: Report of the Surgeon General. Washington, DC, U.S. Department of Health and Human Services, 1980

19. King J, Eiser JR: A strategy for counselling pregnant smokers. Journal of Health Education 40:66-68, 1981

20. Streissguth AP, Landesman-Dwyer S, Martin JC, et al: Teratogenic effects of alcohol in humans and laboratory animals. Science 209:353-361, 1980

21. Sokol RJ, Miller SI, Reed G: Alcohol abuse during pregnancy: an epidemiological study. Alcoholism 4:135-145, 1980
22. Streissguth AP, Darby BL, Barr HM, et al: Comparison of drinking and smoking patterns during pregnancy over a six year interval. Am J Obstet Gynecol 145:716-724 1983
23. Hinman RA: Measles and rubella in adolescents and young adults. Hosp Pract 17:137-146, 1982
24. Adams MM, Erickson JD, Layde PM, et al: Down's syndrome: recent trends in the United States. JAMA 246:758-760, 1984
25. Adams MM, Oakley JP, Marks JS: Maternal age and births in the 1980s. JAMA 247:493-494, 1982
26. National Center for Health Statistics: Advance report of final natality statistics, 1982. Monthly Vital Statistics Report 33 (6), 1984
27. Laurence KM: Effect of early surgery for spina bifida cystica on survival and quality of life. Lancet 1:301-304, 1974
28. Tew BJ, Laurence KM, Payne H, et al: Marital stability following the birth of a child with spina bifida. Br J Psychiatry 131:79-82, 1977
29. Scriver CR: Phenylketonuria: epitome of human biochemical genetics. N Engl J Med 303:1336-1342, 1980
30. Dussault JH: Modification of a screening program for neonatal hypothyroidism. Pediatrics 92:274-277, 1978
31. Grover R, Wethers D, Shahadi S, eat al: Evaluation of the expanded newborn screening program in New York City. Pediatrics 61:740-749, 1978
32. Lenke RR, Levy H: Maternal phenylketonuria and hyperphenylalaninemia: an international survey of the outcome of treated and untreated pregnancies. N Engl J Med 303:1202-1208, 1980
33. Centers for Disease Control: Years of potential life lost, deaths, and death rates. Morbidity and Mortality Weekly Report 34:139, 1985
34. Walton WW: An evaluation of the poison prevention packaging act. Pediatrics 69:363-370, 1982
35. Needleman H, Gunnoe C, Leviton A, et al: Psychological performance of children with elevated lead levels. N Engl J Med 300:689-695, 1979
36. Centers for Disease Control: Blood lead levels in U.S. population. Morbidity and Mortality Weekly Report 31:132-134, 1982
37. Advisory Committee on Immunization Practices: Polysaccharide vaccine for prevention of hemophilus influenzae type b disease. Morbidity and Mortality Weekly Report 34:201-205, 1985
38. Brown GW, Harris T: Social Origins of Depression. New York, Free Press, 1978

39. Hardy JB: Birth weight and subsequent physical and intellectual development. N Engl J Med 289:973-974, 1973
40. Furstenberg FF: The social consequences of teenage parenthood. Fam Plann Perspect 8:148-164, 1976
41. Taylor B, Wadsworth J, Butler NR: Teenage mothering, admission to hospital, and accidents during the first years. Arch Dis Child 58:6-11, 1983
42. Forssman H, Thuwe I: 120 children born after application for therapeutic abortion was refused. Acta Psychiatr Scand 42:71-88, 1966
43. Matejeck Z, Dytrych A, Schuller V: Children from unwanted pregnancies. Acta Psychiatr Scand 57:67-90, 1978
44. Sachs BP, Layde PM, Rubin GL, et al: A review of the economic evidence on prevention. Medical Care 18:473-484, 1980
45. Grossman M, Jacobowitz S: Variations in infant mortality rates among counties in the United States. Demography 18:695-713, 1981
46. Ory HW: Mortality associated with fertility and fertility control. Fam Plann Perspect 15:57-63, 1983
47. Daling JR, Emanuel I: Induced abortion and subsequent outcome of pregnancy in a series of American women. N Engl J Med 197:1241-1245, 1977
48. Hogue CJ, Cates W, Tietze C: The effects of induced abortion on subsequent reproduction. Epidemiol Rev 4:66-91 1982
49. Greer RH, Lao S, Lewis CS, et al: Psychosocial consequences of therapeutic abortion. Br J Psychiatry 128:74-79, 1976
50. Jones EF, Forrest JD, Goldman N, et al: Teenage pregnancy in developed countries: determinants and policy implications. Fam Plann Perspect 17:53-63, 1985
51. Eisenberg L, Earls FJ: Poverty, social depreciation and child development, in American Handbook of Psychiatry (Volume 6). Edited by Hamburg DA. New York, Basic Books, 1975
52. Rutter M, Madge N: Cycles of Disadvantage. London, Heinemann Educational Books, 1976
53. Consortium for Longitudinal Studies: As the Twig is Bent: Lasting Effects of Preschool Programs. Hillsdale, NJ, Erlbaum, 1983
54. Berruetta-Clement JR, Schweinhart LJ, Barnett WS, et al: Changed Lives: The Effects of the Perry Preschool Program on Youths Through Age 19 (Monograph No. 8). Ypsilanti, High/Scope Press, 1984
55. Jordan TJ, Grallo R, Deutsch M, Deutsch CP: Long-term effects of early enrichment: a twenty year-perspective on persistence and change. Am J Community Psychol 13:393-415,

1985
56. Rutter M, Maughan B, Mortimore P, et al: Fifteen Thousand Hours: Secondary Schools and Their Effects on Children. Cambridge, MA, Harvard University Press, 1979
57. Turco RP, Toon OB, Ackerman TP, et al: Nuclear winter: global consequences of multiple nuclear explosions. Science 222:1283-1292, 1983
58. Ehrlich PR, Harte J, Harwell MA, et al: Long-term biological consequences of nuclear war. Science 222:1293-1299, 1983
59. Keller B: As arms buildup eases, U.S. tries to take stock. New York Times, May 14, 1985
60. Eisenberg L: Rudolf Karl Virchow, where are you now that we need you? Am J Med 77:524-532, 1984
61. Miller CA: Infant mortality in the U.S. Sci Am 253:31-37, 1985

4

Possible Prevention Strategies for Depression in Children and Adolescents

Joaquim Puig-Antich, M.D.

4

Possible Prevention Strategies for Depression in Children and Adolescents

For a group of disorders of recent recognition, it may be premature to talk about prevention, since no studies have been carried out yet to indicate if there are any effective prophylactic interventions, and therefore no data are available.

Most systematic research studies of the affective disorders of children and adolescents have been initiated within the last decade. The accumulated knowledge, although substantial (1), is probably not sufficient to describe the nature of the disorders and pose research questions for specific and meaningful prevention strategies. Nevertheless, solid leads do exist. Therefore, it is timely to determine what the work already done tells us about possible strategies for prevention of affective disorders in young people.

Before embarking on such an exploration, one has to ask, Is it worthwhile to prevent such episodes? Rutter (2) pointed out the myths and unknowns surrounding the subject of prevention of child and adolescent disorders. Secondary and tertiary prevention make a lot of sense clinically because of the accumulating handicaps these chronic conditions engender. Because we are so far away from effective primary prevention strategies and the ethical problems are so complex, tertiary prevention may be of extreme scientific interest. However, it has limited immediate applicability, except for focusing our attention more on screening for the first signs of disorder in the children at risk. Although wide application of preventive strategies does not always follow once we learn what we can do (2), few would dispute that such knowledge acquisition is the first order of business.

CONTINUITY OF AFFECTIVE DISORDERS
ACROSS THE LIFESPAN

The attempt to devise potential prophylactic strategies is made easier by the substantial evidence supporting the continuity between the affective disorders classically described in adults and those of childhood or adolescent onset. The hypothesis of continuity across the life span is based on three different sets of comparative data on depression across the life span: 1) natural history and follow up, 2) familial aggregation, and 3) psychobiological markers.

Natural History

Long-term follow-up studies of affective disorder in youth have not been conducted for a sufficient length of time to allow the subjects to reach adulthood. To date, the follow-up studies indicate continued liability for affective disorder as predicted. The current follow-up studies of adult depressive illness (3, 4, 5), adolescent depressive illness (6), and prepubertal depressive illness (7, 8) all show similar life table curves. Although final proof of continuity between child and adult depressive illness is not in from the follow-up data, the similarity of courses and outcomes among childhood-onset, adolescent-onset, and adult-onset affective disorders provides substantial support for the hypothesis of continuity across the life span.

A chronic course for prepubertal affective disorder is the rule; it is also, but somewhat less often, the case in adolescence. With prepubertal onset, spontaneous recovery from either dysthymic disorder or major depressive disorder takes place between one and five years. Nevertheless, the appearance of new episodes before five years after the previous episode is also the rule in at least three-quarters of the patients (8).

Prepubertal depressive illness may have a frequent bipolar outcome in adolescence. Although prepubertal forms of bipolar illness are relatively rare, they do occur and are characterized by elation, marked irritability, mixed manic-depressive pictures, and/or rapid cycling. Patients who do not develop their first depressive episode until adolescence are more likely than those with prepubertal onset of affective illness to present episodes with more clearly delineated or acute onset.

Short- and long-term follow-up studies have also shown that affective disorders with childhood or adolescent onset are likely to be recurrent. If early and proper treatment is not forthcoming, considerable short- and long-term difficulties and complications appear, including poor academic achievement, arrest in psychosocial developmental patterns (9-10), persistent negative self-esteem that complicates frequent negative reinforcement, suicide, drug and alcohol abuse as a means of self-treatment (11), and development of conduct disorder (10).

Familial Aggregation Studies

Familial aggregations of studies of child and adolescent affective disorder are of two types: 1) examinations of offspring younger than age 18 from identified adult patients who have an unequivocal unipolar or bipolar affective disorder ("from the top down") (11, 13, 14, and 15) and 2) those in which lifetime prevalence of psychiatric diagnoses is ascertained in first- and second-degree adult relatives of children and adolescents properly diagnosed as bipolar or nonbipolar major depressive disorder ("from the bottom up") (16-19). The consensus from both perspectives is of a familial pattern of incidence: Affective disorders in children, adolescents, and adults tend to cluster in the same families.

Furthermore, among the child, adolescent, and adult probands studied in the familial aggregation studies, age-adjusted morbidity risks for major depressive disorder in the relatives have been lower the older the probands' mean age of onset. This has been apparent even in restricted ranges of age of onset in young adults (20). Therefore, age of onset of affective illness is likely to be inversely correlated with affective density and depth of affective loading of the pedigree (18), which in turn is also directly related to the risk of bipolarity and other affective disorders in the offspring. The more multigenerational the familial loading with affective disorder, the higher the proportion of offspring likely to be affected, the younger their age of onset is likely to be (17), and the more frequently a bipolar outcome is likely to occur (18). Stated more simply, having one depressed parent probably doubles the risk of the offspring developing affective episode before age 18 years, over the risk of the offsprings' developing affective episode before age 18 compared with the risk in children of nonaffected parents. Children with two depressed parents are several times more likely to present an affective disorder during the same period (21).

Furthermore, familial aggregation in patients with age of onset over 45 years of age does not differ significantly from that of never-depressed controls (20).

Familial aggregation studies support strongly the continuity of child, adolescent, and adult affective disorders. They also suggest that the depth and density of affective loading are probably major causal factors in the development of affective illness in children and adolescents. If affective disorders are the same illness for both age groups, then the evidence supports the importance of genetic factors. Twin and adoption studies of adult affective disorders reveal that evidence of genetic transmissions is stronger for bipolars than for unipolars (22-25). The data also suggest that genetic factors are likely to be more important the younger the age of onset (20).

Psychobiological Markers

The data for biological markers found abnormal during a depressive episode in children and in adolescents are consistent with the age influences observed in the same markers in adults from age 18 to old age. This is especially true in the area of sleep electroencephalograms (EEGs), which we will take as an illustrative example. Despite frequent subjective sleep complaints, prepubertal children do not show polysomnographic abnormalities during a major depressive episode (26, 27). Although unexpected, this finding is consistent with the influence of age on sleep EEG correlates of major depressive disorder in adult years, which is that the younger the patient, the less abnormal the sleep EEG is likely to be. Sleep EEG is also basically normal in adolescent depressives (Goetz et al. in press 23A) except in the 18- to 20-year-old range (28), when rapid eye movement (REM) abnormalities in the expected direction begin to occur. Therefore, sleep EEG abnormalities during a major depressive episode in adults may be secondary to an interaction between depression and age (26).

In contrast to the lack of polysomnographic findings during illness, after sustained recovery from the depressive syndrome and in a drug-free state, prepubertal children show shortened REM latency (29). The evidence on REM latency in fully recovered adult depressives is still contradictory, except regarding the presence of a higher sensitivity to muscarinic receptor agonists manifested by an excessive tendency to REM period advance (30, 31).

Some neuroendocrine markers, especially growth hormone secretion, are also found to be abnormal in fully recovered drug-free prepubertal children with major depression (32-35). Such markers, which become or remain abnormal upon recovery, may be true trait markers or may be markers of a past episode. If the abnormality was present before the first depressive episode, then the neuroendocrine markers may be true trait markers. If the marker is manifested only after the first episode is over, then it is a marker of a past episode. What is exciting about these findings is that a true trait marker has the potential to reflect genetic predisposition to these disorders much earlier than the clinical phenotype (the depressive episodes themselves) and therefore is a more sensitive indicator of predisposition. As such, trait markers could be very helpful in conducting high-risk and prophylactic studies and in ascertaining mode of transmission of the affective disorders in informative pedigrees.

PREVENTION

Keeping in mind the three sets of comparative data from natural history and follow-up studies, familial aggregation, and psychobiological marker studies, we can now consider different levels of prophylactic interventions that could be tested. They are discussed in two groups: primary prevention and secondary and tertiary prevention.

Primary Prevention

Attempts to prevent the disorder before it can occur and thus decrease its incidence and prevalence can be conceivably made in four different ways:

Cohort Effects. One approach is to establish the reasons for the existence of what appears to be a cohort effect in both suicide and affective illness. Results of several studies (20, 21) have indicated that during the last few decades the prevalence of affective illness has been increasing from generation to generation. The problem in interpreting such data is that most of the assessments done for the older generation have been done at the present time and are basically retrospective. Thus, there may be an ascertainment bias, which may also be due to differential mortality rates. Nevertheless, some of these data do not seem to be subject to the same sources of bias. For example, the incidence of suicide in adolescents appears to be rising on a year-to-year basis, and this seems to be even more true in young adults (36). If this is truly a cohort effect, it would suggest that there is some environmental circumstance or complex of circumstances causing it. If so, discovering such causal factors could materially prevent at least a further rise in the incidence and prevalence of these disorders. Without such knowledge, interventions are bound to fail.

Genetic Counseling. A second approach is genetic counseling. Although not final, the degree of concordance among several studies of familial aggregation is quite impressive, in spite of the substantial variability in methods of selection of the probands, as described above. Therefore, genetic counseling may have a role in preventing affective illness of very early onset. But is unlikely to be of any importance in preventing affective illness beginning after age 45.

Trait Markers. Third, the exciting possibility of the existence of trait markers in prepubertal major depression needs to be explored. Such trait markers would remain abnormal in recovery and not be related to how long after the episode they are tested (within a range of one to four months). Their discovery would open up new vistas for the possibility of the existence of a true trait marker that would precede the onset of the first episode of affective illness. If such true trait markers were found, they would enable researchers to identify which offspring of at-risk families (those with high familial aggregation of affective illness) will be ill during the formative years. Furthermore, together with chromosomal linkage analyses using the new DNA polymorphism techniques, such markers would be very useful for the eventual determination of the familial modes of transmission of these disorders.

Identification of Psychosocial Risk. The final potential strategy of primary prevention is identification of psychosocial risk. Beginning explorations of the possible roles of nongenetic factors in affective illness in children, although not definitive, have exhibited remarkably uniform negative results. Little evidence at present suggests that marital status of the parent, marital functioning, size of sibships, socioeconomic status, familial constellation, or structure play much of a role in the occurrence of depressive disorders in children. An exception is Weissman's study (13), in which divorce was associated with a slightly increased rate of affected offspring.

Nevertheless, it has to be said that the definitions and specificity of psychosocial risk are not very satisfactory. One has to begin with the hypothesis that the factors relevant to the psychosocial risk for development of affective disorder in children may not necessarily be the same psychosocial risk factors that have been found to be associated to the development of general child psychiatric disorders (2).

In my opinion, it is likely that among preschoolers in whom depressive-like clinical presentations are beginning to be described, the role of environmental influences will receive more experimental support. These factors may vary substantially with development, from preschool to young adulthood. If so it will be crucial to differentiate children who have a high genetic risk for affective disorder from those whose depressive pictures are mostly secondary to relatively drastic psychosocial familial circumstances without familial aggregation for affective disorders and who therefore may constitute true phenocopies. Prior research has suggested that severe distortions in parenting and family function are associated with the development of conduct disorder and antisocial personality (37) but not necessarily with the development of affective illness.

Secondary and Tertiary Prevention

Secondary prevention aims at the early identification and rapid treatment of a disorder. The goal is to decrease the prevalence in lieu of the incidence. Tertiary prevention aims to prevent chronicity by the effective treatment of the main disorder and the prevention and/or treatment of secondary complications. Although easy to distinguish in theory, secondary and tertiary preventions tend to become intertwined when one considers very early onset affective illness. Improper assessment and misdiagnosis of affective disorder in children referred to child mental health services is a major obstacle to effective treatment and secondary and tertiary prevention. In the past 15 to 20 years there has been increasing evidence that symptom-focused interviews are not only reliable but also valid in children of school age (38-41). They are probably the most important component in the diagnostic evaluation of a child in whom affective disorder is suspected. Yet this evidence has not been fully incorporated into child psychiatric practice and has been incorporated even less into the practice of other mental health professionals. For many years, "play interviews" have dominated child psychiatric practice. Play interviews are the proper format from which to elicit worries and symbolic constellations, but they are not helpful in eliciting psychiatric symptoms upon which we base modern child psychiatric diagnosis. Simply said, the child professional can play with the child from now until doomsday, but unless the proper questions are asked few or none of the symptoms the child is suffering from will be discovered. Another obstacle today is that treatment of child and adolescent affective disorder is in fact in its infancy. There is no final proof of the efficacy of any of the antidepressants. Among prepubertal children with major depression (and probably dysthymia), there is substantial evidence that antidepressant medication may be effective, because of the relationship found in at least two different studies between IMI and DMI steady-state plasma levels and clinical response (42, 43), which are similar to what is found in the older adult patients (44, 45). But there is as yet no final convincing evidence on differential efficacy of tricyclic antidepressants versus placebo in prepubertal depression. At present two studies are ongoing to test this point further.

For adolescents, the picture appears to be somewhat different. Ryan et al. (46) found a low response rate (44 percent) and no relationship between outcome and plasma levels in 34 adolescent nonbipolar major depressive disorder patients treated with imipramine for six weeks (mean dose = 26 mg/day). Other types of antidepressants should be tested. On the other hand, lithium seems to be as effective in treatment and future prevention of adolescent-onset bipolar illness as it is in adults. However, again, no controlled studies of lithium are available for this age group. The natural course of the disorder, as demonstrated by Kovacs (7, 8) and by Strober (6), clearly justifies aggressive psychopharmacological and other treatment.

Finally, no controlled studies have been conducted on psychosocial interventions in child or adolescent depressive disorders. Recently, functional impairment associated with depressive disorder in childhood was found to extend to almost all areas of the child psychosocial world, including school performance, peer relationships, and family relations (9). Children's relationships with their parents, peers, and siblings were markedly abnormal during the major depressive episode. In contrast, the rate of marital breakups or the quality of marital relationships among the parents of depressed children was no different from those of control families. On sustained recovery from the depressive episode (10), the children's relationships slowly improved, whereas no changes could be detected in the parental marital relationship. Generally, considerable impairment in social skills still exists after 4 months of total recovery from major depression in prepubertal children. Such hesitance of psychosocial impairment is probably related to the duration of the prior episode of depression/dysthymia.

Child psychotherapy as generally practiced does not appear to be very effective in treating a depressive symptomatology or any other aspect of the child psychopathology if the youngster is severely depressed (7, 10, 46). On the basis of clinical experience with affectively disordered children, it seems sensible to defer a decision of psychotherapeutic intervention until after the youngster has recovered from a major depressive disorder. The best indication of psychosocial treatment is a lack of spontaneous gradual improvement in social functioning and relationships after remission of the affective picture. The accuracy of this clinical impression should be tested in future controlled studies.

Complications of Very Early Onset Affective Disorders

The complications that can arise in a very early onset affective illness should be considered in prophylaxis research on these disorders. There are two types of complications:

Complications Due to the Nature of the Episode. Acute complications may arise because of the nature and severity of the affective illness. Suicidal behavior, the extreme irritability of some bipolar forms, mixed bipolar disorders, the presence of dysthymia, the presence psychotic symptoms frequently with suicidal command auditory hallucinations, and the often massive psychosocial deficits during the episode need different types of protective intervention during acute treatment. These complications usually respond in parallel to the severity of the affective episode.

Complications Due to Associated Characteristics. Another set of complications comes from the presence of associated characteristics that appear to be somewhat unique to depressed children and adolescents with major depressive disorder. They rarely present a "pure" clinical picture. The two main symptom complexes associated with affective illness in these age groups are neurotic symptoms or disorders, especially separation anxiety, and conduct disorder.

Separation anxiety of a moderate or severe degree appears in approximately one-third of the children (47) and probably in a somewhat smaller proportion of adolescents. In older adolescents, full-fledged panic attacks are common. Associated fears or phobias with a relatively high degree of general or background anxiety have been found in a significant proportion of children. There is little evidence today that the presence of this anxiety symptom makes a difference in treatment, because it usually responds to antidepressant medications.

Although obsessive compulsive symptoms occur in only a minority of depressive/dysthymic youngsters, a majority of patients younger than age 18 with obsessive compulsive disorder have suffered or do suffer from episodes of major depression (48). Treatment of depression frequently is not sufficient for full recovery from obsessive compulsive symptoms, which may need to be addressed separately.

A coexisting diagnosis of conduct disorder with that of major depression or dysthymia is rather frequent particularly among boys (12). Children whose primary diagnosis is conduct disorder often are miserable. In some of these children, secondary episodes of major depression of dysthymia develop. There is little evidence to show that successful treatment of their secondary affective illness has any bearing on the severity of course of the primary conduct disorder.

In contrast, in cases of primary depression or dysthymia with a secondary diagnosis of conduct disorder, successful treatment of the affective illness is likely to be followed by the waning of conduct disorder behavioral patterns (12). This course mirrors the chronology of the onset of the episode, in which the affective illness triggered the onset of secondary conduct disorder. These observations underscore the critical importance of proper semi-structured assessment of the child's mental status for treatment planning, because there is little to offer as effective treatment for moderate to severe primary conduct disorder. In children with depressive disorders, predisposed to conduct disorders, the affective illness may lower the threshold for the eruption of conduct behaviors. Furthermore, given the long duration and high frequency of recurring episodes of depression among youth, it is also likely that the associated secondary conduct disorder, feeding on its own circle of negative social reinforcement, will increasingly dominate the clinical picture in untreated cases. Thus, the development of conduct disorder in an affectively ill child should be considered a risk factor for future progression to antisocial personality, alcoholism, substance abuse, and general social maladjustment in adolescent and adulthood. It is therefore logical that treatment should not only be directed to the present episode or the disorder but should also be instituted as early as possible for all subsequent episodes, in order to avoid secondary complications of very early onset affective illness.

Compared with adult-onset affective illness, childhood affective illness tends to follow a generally more insidious onset and chronic course. Familial aggregation displays higher density for affective disorders and alcoholism and is more likely to develop secondary complications of accumulating psychosocial deficits, conduct disorder, alcoholism, substance abuse, and antisocial personality traits in both the short run and the long run. Furthermore, among adolescents it is not infrequent to see alcohol and drug abuse that, until detoxification has occurred, mask an affective illness. This is especially common among first-degree relatives (offspring or siblings) of bipolar adults (11) and has fundamental implications for proper treatment.

The evidence indicates that major depression or dysthymia in youngsters predicts future affective episodes. Depressive episodes in childhood tend to be longer and more confined for a long time before the patient or the family accept their presence and request treatment again. Affective episodes involve severe functional impairment and disability as well as a marked decrease in the quality of life. In some cases the patient's life is in danger. These problems are likely to be cumulative in youngsters and to worsen with increasing duration of the episodes. They probably make full recovery from affective and nonaffective aspects of an episode progressively more difficult to achieve over time.

Given these factors, the long-term aid should be to keep the patient as free as possible of periods of affective illness. The safest way to achieve this deal for nonbipolar children is to educate them and their families to recognize the onset of episodes and report them immediately to their treating physician. Thus the treatment of very early onset affective illness should be viewed always as a long-term partnership between the patient, the family, and the physician. The child and the parents should be informed that the child is more likely than others to develop subsequent episodes of depression and that as soon as symptoms recur, if they indeed do, the doctor should be contacted. With the aid of such a program these children can lead normal lives and develop without any more obstacles than their peers have. Such a partnership constitutes an excellent example of secondary and tertiary prevention.

REFERENCES

1. Puig-Antich J: Affective disorders in children and adolescents, in Kaplan HI, Saddock BJ (eds.): Comprehensive Textbook of Psychiatry: Volume IV. Williams & Wilkins, Baltimore, 1984
2. Rutter M: Prevention of children's psychosocial disorders. Pediatrics, 70:883-894, 1982
3. Keller MB, Shapiro RW, Lavori PW, et al: Recovery in major depressive disorder. Arch Gen Psychiatry 39:905-910, 1982
4. Keller MB, Shapiro RW, Lavori PW, et al: Relapse in major depressive disorder. Arch Gen Psychiatry 39:911-920, 1982
5. Keller MB, Lavori PW, Lewis CE, et al: Predictors of relapse in major depressive disorder. JAMA 250:199-204, 1984
6. Strober M: Follow-up of Adolescent Affective Disorder Patients. Paper presented at the annual meeting of the American Psychiatric Association, New York, May 1983
7. Kovacs M, Feinberg TL, Crouse-Novak MA, et al: Depressive disorders in childhood. 1. A longitudinal prospective study of characteristics and recovery. Arch Gen Psychiatry 41:219-239, 1984
8. Kovacs M, Feinberg TL, Crouse-Novak MA, et al: Depressive disorders in childhood. 2. A longitudinal study of the risk for a subsequent major depression. Arch Gen Psychiatry 41:643-649, 1984

9. Puig-Antich J, Lukens E, Davies M, et al: Psychosocial functioning in prepubertal major depressive disorders. 1. Interpersonal relationships during the depressive episode. Arch Gen Psychiatry 42:500-507, 1985

10. Puig-Antich J, Lukens E, Davies M, et al: Psychosocial functioning in prepubertal major depressive disorders. 2. Interpersonal relationships after sustained recovery from the affective episode. Arch Gen Psychiatry 42:511-517, 1985

11. Akiskal HS, Downs J, Jordan P, et al: Affective disorders in referred children and younger siblings of manic-depressives. Arch Gen Psychiatry 42:996-1003, 1985

12. Puig-Antich J: Major depression and conduct disorder in prepuberty. J Am Acad Child Psychiatry 21:118-128, 1982

13. Weissman MM, Leckman JF, Merikangas KR, et al: Depression and anxiety disorders in parents and children. Arch Gen Psychiatry 41:845-852, 1984

14. Welner Z, Welzer A, McCray MD, et al: Psychopathology in children of inpatients with depression: a controlled study. J Nerv Ment Dis 164:408-413, 1977

15. Gershon ES, McKnew D, Cytryn L, et al: Diagnoses in school-age children of bipolar affective disorder patients and normal controls. J Affective Disord 8:283-291, 1985

16. Puig-Antich J, Goetz D, Davies M, et al: A Controlled Family History Study of Prepubertal Major Depressive Disorder. Paper presented at the annual meeting of the American Academy of Child Psychiatry, San Francisco, CA, October 1982

17. Puig-Antich J, Goetz D, Davies M, et al: A Controlled Family History Study of Adolescent Major Depressive Disorder. Paper presented at the American Academy of Child Psychiatry, 1983

18. Strober M, Carlson G: Bipolar illness in adolescent with major depression. Arch Gen Psychiatry 39:549-558, 1982

19. Strober M, Burroughs J, Salkin B, et al: Ancestral secondary cases of psychiatric illness in adolescents with mania, depression, schizophrenia and conduct disorder. Biol Psychiatry, in press

20. Weissman MM, Wickramaratne P, Merikangas KR, et al: Onset of major depression in early adulthood: increased familial loading and specificity. Arch Gen Psychiatry, in press

21. Gershon ES, Hanovit J, Guroff JJ, et al: A family study of schizoaffective, bipolar II, unipolar, and normal control probands. Arch Gen Psychiatry 39:1157-1167, 1982

22. Gershon ES, Bunney WE Jr, Leckman JF, et al: The inheritance of affective disorders: a review of data and hypotheses. Behav Genet 227-261, 1976

23. Bertelsen A, Harvald B, Hauge M: A Danish twin study of

manic depressive disorder. Br J Psychiatry 130:330-357, 1977
24. Mendlewicz J: Adoption study supporting genetic transmission in manic-depressive illness. Nature 268:327-329, 1977
25. Cadoret RJ, Gorman TW, Heywood E, et al: Genetic and environmental factors in major depression. J Affective Disord 9:155-164, 1985
26. Puig-Antich J, Goetz R, Hanlon C, et al: Sleep architecture and REM sleep measures in prepubertal major depressives during an episode. Arch Gen Psychiatry 39:932-939, 1982
27. Young W, Knowles JB, MacLean AW, et al: The sleep of childhood depressives: comparison with age-matched controls. Biol Psychiatry 17:1163-1168, 1982
28. Lahmeyer HW, Poznanski EO, Bellur SN: EEG sleep in depressed adolescents. Am J Psychiatry 140:1150-1153, 1983
29. Puig-Antich J, Goetz R, Hanlon C, et al: Sleep architecture and REM sleep measures in prepubertal major depressives: studies during recovery from a major depressive episode in a drug-free state. Arch Gen Psychiatry 40:187-192, 1983
30. Sitaram M, Nurnberger JI, Gershon ES, et al: Faster cholinergic REM sleep induction in euthymic patients with primary affective illness. Science 208:200-201, 1980
31. Dube S, Kumar N, Ettedgui E, et al: Cholinergic REM induction response: separation of anxiety and depression. Biol Psychiatry 20:408-418, 1985
32. Puig-Antich J, Novacenko H, Davies M, et al: Growth hormone secretion in prepubertal major depressive children. 1. Response to insulin induced hypoglycemia. Final Report. Arch Gen Psychiatry 41:455-460, 1984
33. Puig-Antich J, Goetz R, Davies M, et al: Growth hormone secretion in prepubertal major depressive children. 2. Sleep related plasma concentrations during a depressive episode. Arch Gen Psychiatry 41:463-466, 1984
34. Puig-Antich J, Davies M, Novacenko H, et al: Growth hormone secretion in prepubertal major depressive children. 3. Response to insulin-induced hypoglycemia in a drug-free, fully recovered clinical state. Arch Gen Psychiatry 41:471-475, 1984
35. Puig-Antich J, Goetz R, Davies M, et al: Growth hormone secretion in prepubertal major depressive children. 4. Sleep related plasma concentrations in a drug-free fully recovered clinical state. Arch Gen Psychiatry 41:479-483, 1984
36. Shaffer D: Depression and suicide in children and adolescents, in Child and Adolescent Psychiatry: Modern Approaches (Second Edition). Edited by Rutter M, Hersov L. Boston, Blackwell, 1985

37. Rutter M: Maternal deprivation reconsidered. J Psychosom Res 16:241-250, 1972
38. Herjanic B, Herjanic M, Brown F, et al: Are children reliable reporters? Journal of the Association of Child Psychology and Psychiatry 3:41-48, 1975
39. Rutter M, Graham P: The reliability and validity of the psychiatric assessment of the child. 1. Interview with the child. Br J Psychiatry 114:563-579, 1968
40. Poznanski EO, Grossman JA, Buchsbaum Y, et al: Preliminary studies of the reliability and validity of the Children's Depression Rating Scale. J Am Acad Child Psychiatry 23:191-197, 1984
41. Chambers WJ, Puig-Antich J, Hirsch M, et al: The assessment of affective disorders in children and adolescents by semi-structured interview: test-retest reliability of the K-SADS-P. Arch Gen Psychiatry 42:696-702, 1985
42. Preskorn S, Weller EB, Weller RA: Depression in children: relationship between plasma imipramine levels and response. J Clin Psychiatry 43:450-453, 1982
43. Puig-Antich J, Perel J, Lupatkin W, et al: Imipramine in prepubertal major depression. Arch Gen Psychiatry, in press
44. Glassman AH, Perel JM, Shostak M, et al: Clinical implications of imipramine plasma levels for depressive illness. Arch Gen Psychiatry 34:197-204, 1977
45. Reisby N, Gram LF, Bech P, et al: Imipramine: clinical effects and pharmacokinetic variability. Psychopharm 54:263-272, 1977
46. Ryan ND, Puig-Antich J, Cooper T, et al: Imipramine in adolescent major depression: plasma level and clinical response. Acta Psychiatr Scand, in press
47. Puig-Antich J, Rabinovich H: Relationship between affective and anxiety disorders of childhood, in Anxiety Disorders of Childhood. Edited by Gittelman R. New York, Guilford Press, in press
48. Rapoport JL, Elkins R, Langer DH, et al: Childhood obsessive-compulsive disorder. Am J Psychiatry 138:1545-1554, 1981

5

Prevention of Schizophrenia: What Do We Know?

Michael J. Goldstein, Ph.D.

Joan R. Asarnow, Ph.D.

5

Prevention of Schizophrenia: What Do We Know?

In 1980 the National Institute of Mental Health (NIMH) Office of Prevention sponsored a conference entitled "Preventive Interventions in Schizophrenia: Are We Ready?" (1). The general consensus of the meeting, at which many leading scholars presented papers, was that because we did not have clear-cut methods for identifying individuals at risk for the disorder, large-scale preventive intervention efforts for schizophrenia were not justified at that time. Conference participants were more encouraging about prevention-oriented research to evaluate the alterability of selected attributes of individuals of family units thought to be at risk for a schizophrenic disorder.

Although a cautionary attitude regarding large-scale preventive intervention programs is still desirable, it is now possible to take a more positive outlook toward prevention of schizophrenia. There are two reasons for this. First, a number of studies of children at risk for schizophrenia are nearing completion and identify vulnerability markers for the disorder's being a probable outcome. For example, at a recent (April 1985) NIMH conference entitled "Risk Factors in Schizophrenia: Current Status and Future Directions," the leading investigators of these longitudinal prospective studies reported similar findings in terms of documentation of attributes of children at risk for schizophrenia, as well as family attributes associated with offspring risk for psychiatric disorder. These cross study results are impressive.

Second, it has become clear since 1980 that the conceptual meaning of prevention of schizophrenia should include recognition of the continuity between efforts designed to prevent the onset of schizophrenia and those designed to prevent reoccurrence. Before we begin discussing prevention of schizophrenia, let's consider prevention in general as applied to any major mental disorder, such as schizophrenia, in which a considerable gap exists between birth and onset of the disorder in late adolescence or early adulthood.

PREVENTION: A CONCEPT REVISITED

The ultimate goal of prevention research is to define some forms of intervention that can be applied early in life to inhibit the expression of the disorder during a subsequent life period when an individual is at risk. Although this point has never been made explicit, effective prevention should also minimize the expression of precursor states that antedate, often by many years, the initial onset of the clinical state we call schizophrenia. There are two strategies to this type of prevention: 1) applying some sort of blanket immunity procedure to all individuals in society that can prevent schizophrenia independent of one's liability to the disorder and 2) identifying groups of individuals who are at particularly high risk for the disorder and then targeting preventive interventions.

In the first strategy, we need a clear understanding of the etiology or etiologies of this disorder (or disorders, as is most likely the case) and a mechanism for reversing or inhibiting the underlying pathophysiology and psychopathology. In addition, the agent for application of the immunity would have to be of low risk for all persons, regardless of their liability to the disorder. Obviously, there are many problems with this strategy. We know little about the etiology or etiologies of schizophrenia and thus have few clues to possible generic immunity programs. Thus, there is little potential for such communitywide prevention programs. Undoubtedly, many things could be done to promote higher levels of mental health in the population at large that could also operate to reduce the risk for schizophrenia. These programs may be valuable and justifiable, but they obviously cannot be considered prevention programs targeted specifically for schizophrenia. Also, it is important to recognize that not everyone believes that prevention programs should be targeted specifically to one or another disorder at all (2, 3). General mental health promotion, it is argued, is the best vehicle for preventing a wide spectrum of mental disorders and research aimed at development of specific prevention programs for specific disorders is wasteful.

The alternative to a general blanket immunity program is a strategy in which groups of individuals with particularly high risk

for the disorder are identified and receive targeted preventive interventions. In order for this strategy to succeed, a mechanism to
identify those individuals within high-risk cohorts who are vulnerable to the disorder must be established. For example, if a
cohort is defined as possessing an attribute that identifies excessive risk for schizophrenia, it may not be essential to identify
those individuals within the cohort who are specifically vulnerable
to a schizophrenic disorder. However, if the method of identifying
cohorts at risk for the disorder is of low specificity, then individual markers are needed to detect the vulnerable members
within the cohort. Until quite recently, the only reliable risk
marker for schizophrenia was the presence of a schizophrenic
parent. Family genetic studies have consistently indicated that 10
to 16 percent of the offspring of one schizophrenic parent are at
risk for the disorder. However, it would be difficult to justify extensive prevention efforts for this population since 86 to 90 percent of the cohort are not at risk for the disorder. If the outcome
criteria are broadened to include a wider variety of psychopathological outcomes, the risk among children of schizophrenics is
muc higher and might justify preventive programs for that
population.

Use of prevention programs could be defended if there were
some way of identifying individuals or family units who are particularly vulnerable to the disorder. Indeed, this is a major objective
of what is referred to as high-risk research related to
schizophrenia. In the following section, the strategy underlying
this type of research is reviewed and current findings from
longitudinal prospective studies are summarized.

HIGH-RISK RESEARCH RELATED TO SCHIZOPHRENIA

High-risk research in schizophrenia has its origins in genetics,
developmental psychology, the study of attention and information
processing in experimental psychology, and the measurement of
intrafamilial processes. One thing that high-risk research studies
have in common, however, is that they all involve longitudinal
prospective studies of populations hypothesized to have a higher
risk for schizophrenia than the general population. (Garmezy of-
fers a comprehensive review of high risk research on
schizophrenia [4, 5].) A cohort is studied over time to identify attributes of individuals or family units that are evident prior to
onset of the disorder and identify the individual or family unit as
being at risk. While this is not a necessary characteristic of a vulnerability marker, it is possible that such a marker may reflect an
underlying pathophysiological or psychopathological process that

contributes to the development of a schizophrenic disorder.

Naturally, when a vulnerability marker identifies a potential etiological pathway to the disorder, the implications for preventive intervention are greater than when a vulnerability marker is correlated with the subsequent disorder but bears little or no relationship to etiology. It is not always clearly understood that longitudinal prospective studies are observational, not experimental, and thus merely provide clues to etiology by establishing antecedent-consequence relationships. Such studies cannot serve as tests of causal links. Ironically, only preventive intervention trials, in which we attempt to modify vulnerability markers and observe subsequent rates of disorder, can establish whether the marker itself or the process it reflects identifies causal pathway to the disorder. For this reason, a useful objective for prevention research at the present time is to establish whether vulnerability markers are modifiable and whether such modifications have an impact, in the short term, on the symptoms and cognitive and social functioning of the youngster at risk. A similar question is applicable to vulnerability markers of intrafamilial processes: Can the attribute be modified, and does modification alter the subsequent psychiatric status of offspring within the family?

Most but not all high-risk studies began with the one established risk marker for schizophrenia, that of schizophrenia in a parent. Within the cohort of offspring of schizophrenics, researchers attempted to discriminate those who were vulnerable from those who were not vulnerable to the disorder. Although this is a reasonable strategy, we should keep in mind that only 10 percent of schizophrenic patients have schizophrenic parents. Therefore any vulnerability markers identified within this cohort may not generalize to the larger population of schizophrenics for whom the risk marker of schizophrenic parentage is absent. This is a critical challenge to many of the high-risk studies that trace the developmental history of offspring of schizophrenic parents.

With this caveat in mind, a review of the findings from high-risk studies follows. As we have indicated previously (6), high-risk studies are designed to answer the following questions:

1. Are there early signs or dysfunctions that identify the child or adolescent as being more at risk for schizophrenia than his or her peers?
2. If yes, at what age and in what specific attributes do at-risk children/adolescents differ from their peers?
3. Are the identifying attributes specific to schizophrenia, or do they merely identify a person at risk for severe psychopathology, regardless of its form?

4. Are there attributes or intrafamilial processes that discriminate the psychosocial environments of preschizophrenic individuals from those of their peers?

Examination of papers prepared for the Risk Research Consortium sponsored by the NIMH in 1985 permits the formulation of some preliminary answers to these questions. In this formulation, certain things should be kept in mind. First, there is wide variation in subject age at which different high-risk studies were begun: Some began while the subjects were prenatal, whereas others began when the subjects were in adolescence. Different phases of the life span were covered in different studies. In addition, only four of the studies were conducted on populations that were close to or well within the risk period for schizophrenia (18 to 45 years of age). For most of the studies, the results reflect attributes that identified a subgroup of the offspring of schizophrenics, but no long-term outcomes are yet available for these subgroups. Nevertheless, we attempted in the present review to investigate whether the attributes found predictive in those studies in which the sample had entered the risk period for schizophrenia parallel the attributes found in subsamples identified as deviant at a younger age.

In a sense, our summary of recurrent findings across the studies is based on some questionable assumptions. Perhaps the most questionable is whether a series of discrete studies, each of which covers only a portion of the life span, can be integrated into a longitudinal model for the development of schizophrenia. However, we think the provocation of further thought about preventive efforts is worth the risk of hypothesizing longitudinal trends from segments of different short-term longitudinal studies.

Table 1 presents the most robust findings we observed across the 23 studies. Each finding represents a statistically significant finding based on an intergroup comparison. However, we did not evaluate the power of the findings in discriminating between groups. This is obviously the next important step in evaluating the sensitivity and specificity of any marker of vulnerability to schizophrenia.

FINDINGS FROM HIGH-RISK STUDIES IN SCHIZOPHRENIA

In terms of the first of the aforementioned four questions to which high-risk studies attempt to provide answers, the answer is yes there clearly are early signs or dysfunctions that identify at-risk children and adolescents (see Table 1). Numerous differences were found that discriminated children of schizophrenic parents

Table 1. Characteristics of High-Risk Children During Five Life Stages in 23 High-Risk Projects

Life Stage	Neurointegrative Functioning	Social Functioning	Symptoms	Family Stressors
Conception to infancy Prenatal				Maternal stress (CD, D-OB, FW, P, SE, RLS, B-R) Maternal risk taking (RLS, SW, P, E)
Perinatal	Small for gestational age; low ponderal index (weight-to-length ratio) (SW) Low birth weight (JIDS, E, RIS)			
Infancy (to age 2)	Abnormal motor and sensory functioning (NY-F, D-OB, SW, IS, JIDS, P, RLS) High or variable sensitivity to sensory stimulation (NY-F, SW, IS, RLS) Abnormal growth patterns (NY-F, P) Short attention span (D) Low IQ (E)	Difficult temperament (SW) Passive, low energy, quiet (D, NY-F) Inhibited, less spontaneous, imitative, expressive (B-G, P, E) Absence of fear of strangers (SW) Low communicative competence (E)		Nonoptimal maternal care (P, RLS, B-G, SW, E, NY-F) Anxious attachment to mother (SW) High activity level in mother-child interaction (E)

Early childhood (ages 2 to 4)	Low reactivity (RLS) Poor gross and fine motor coordination (NCPP-H) Inconsistent performance on cognitive tests (NCPP-H)	Depression (RLS) Angry & hostile disposition (E) Low expressed negative affect (E) Anxiety (E) Schizoid behavior (emotionally flat, withdrawn, distractable, passive, irritable, and negativistic) (NCPP-H, NY-F)		Parental separation during first five years of life (boys only, D) Negative family environment (RLS, URCAFS, E, NY-F)
Middle childhood	Indices of neurological impairment (poor fine motor coordination, balance, sensory perceptual signs, delayed motor development) (IS, NY-F, NY-E, NCPP-H, D-OB, NCPP-R) Attentional impairment under overload conditions (MN, NY-E, SB)	Poor affective control (emotional instability, aggressive, disruptive, hyperactive, impulsive) (SB, NCPP-R, NCPP-H, NY-E, NY-F, IS) Poor interpersonal relationships (MN, SB-girls only, NY-F, IS) Immature (fearful, inhibited, withdrawn (MN, NCPP-R, SB, MA—girls only, NY-F, IS)	Cognitive slippage, disturbance (SB, St. L) Mixed internalizing externalizing symptoms (SB) Attention deficit disorder-like (IS) More disturbed (SW) More childhood disorders (conduct disorder, attention deficit disorder, developmental disorders) (NY-E)	Death of a parent (MA) Low rates of interaction and unbalanced interaction (URCAFS) Mothers show lax discipline (SB) Fathers unaccepting and uninvolved (SB) Poor family relationships (SB) Marital discord (SB) Child shows performance deficits under conditions of

Table 1. Characteristics of High-Risk Children During Five Life Stages in 23 High-Risk Projects (*continued*)

Life Stage	Neurointegrative Functioning	Social Functioning	Symptoms	Family Stressors
		Low cognitive and social competence (URCAFS, SB, IS)		response-contingent social reinforcement by mother (URCAFS)
		Poor attention in school (IS)		Negative family environment (NY-F)
Adolescence	Indices of neurological impairment (poor motor coordination, balance, sensory perceptual signs) (IS, NY-E)	Poor affective control (D, NY-E, St. L, UCLA, IS)	Severe but nonpsychotic behavioral disturbance (UCLA)	Negative family environment (F-T, UCLA, NY-F)
	Attentional impairment under overload condition (NY-E, MW)	Poor interpersonal relationships (D, NY-E, MW, St. L, UCLA, IS)		Parental communication deviance (UCLA)
	Lower IQ (St. L, SB, D, IS)	Poor school adjustment (D, NY-E, MW, NY-F)		Child shows failure to inhibit negative affect in family interaction (UCLA)
	Drop in Comprehension test score of WISC-R between 10 and 15 years of age (2–7 points, NY-F)			
	Inability to use low meaning cues on Referential Communication Task (SB)			

| Early adulthood | Poor performance on WAIS Digit Span and Arithmetic subtests (IS) | Poor social adjustment (IS) | High scores on Perceptual Ab-erration-Magical Ideation scales (for males, high concurrent scores on impulsive nonconformity scale are associated with increased rates of schizotypal symptoms; for females, high concurrent scores on social anhedonia scale are associated with increased rate of schizotypal symptoms) (W) | Negative family environment (F-T) |

Note. General stressors were found to be characteristic of high-risk children in two life stages: In the perinatal stage, delivery complications were found (RLS, P, D, F-W); and in the early childhood stage, institutionalization was found to be a characteristic (D, boys only). B-G = Boston (Grunebaum); B-R = Boston-Ragins; D = Danish-Mednick et al.; D-OB = Danish-Mednick and Schulsinger; E = Emory University-Goodman; F-W = Finland-Wrede; F-T = Finland-Tienari; IS = Israel-Marcus and Rosenthal; JIDS = Jerusalem-Marcus and Auerbach; MA = Massachusetts-Watt; MN = Minnesota-Garmezy et al.; MW = McMaster Waterloo-Asarnow et al.; NCPP-H = National Institute of Neurological and Communicative Diseases and Stroke Perinatal Project (NCPP)-Hanson et al.; NCPP-R = NCPP-Rieder et al.; NY-E = New York-Erlenmeyer-Kimling and Cornblatt; NY-F = New York-Fish; P = Pittsburgh-Schacter and Ragins; RLS = Rochester-Sameroff et al.; SB = Stony Brook-Weintraub and Neale; St. L. = St. Louis-Worland; SW = Sweden-McNeil and Kaij; UCLA = Los Angeles-Goldstein and Rodnick; URCAFS = Rochester-Wynne et al.; W = Wisconsin-Chapman and Chapman. In the D, JIDS, NY-E, and UCLA studies, sample is in risk period for schizophrenia.

from control children. It should be pointed out that not all off-spring of schizophrenics reflected these group trends. Typically, it was only a subset of individuals who appeared deviant, a fact consistent with the expectation of a variable genetic predisposition to the disorder. It should also be noted that the magnitude of the differences are a function of which comparison group was used. When offspring of nonpsychiatric groups were the sole comparison group, differentiation was much sharper than when offspring of parents with another psychiatric disorder (for example, depression) were contrasted.

Although group differences are apparent across the life span, it may be more meaningful for estimating likely targets for prevention to concentrate on which attributes are observable at which developmental stage, the second question that high-risk research attempts to answer. For coherency, we present the findings for a) conception through infancy, b) early childhood, c) middle childhood, and d) adolescence. (Findings for early adulthood, which are presented in Table 1, are not discussed here; the reader is referred to [6].) Again, we are not following a single cohort throughout these life stages but instead are trying to recreate longitudinal patterns from a series of studies limited in overlap with one another from one time period to another.

Prenatal Through Infancy (Conception to Age 2)

At least nine studies covered the prenatal through infancy periods. The findings suggest that some children of schizophrenics are subject to identifiable stressful circumstances and show deviant behavior patterns in the earliest stages of life. Many of the variables characterizing children of schizophrenics appeared to be nonspecific factors associated with severity and chronicity of parental illness or low socioeconomic status. For example, schizophrenic women, as well as women with histories of other psychiatric disorders, were found to experience more stress during pregnancy and be more likely to engage in risk-increasing behaviors. Women with severe psychiatric disorders, including schizophrenia, were likely to report that their pregnancy was unplanned and undesired; expressed fear about pregnancy (7); reported physical discomfort (8); and experienced anxiety, anger, and depression (9, 10).

Low levels of social support were also found for pregnant women with histories of psychiatric disturbance. Such women were more frequently unmarried; when they were married, they tended to have poor marital relationships and/or husbands who expressed negative attitudes toward the pregnancy (7, 8, 11-15).

Risk-increasing behaviors such as medication use (10, 14) and heavy smoking and drinking (7, 9) were also relatively common during the pregnancies of schizophrenic women. Perhaps related to these risk and stress factors, prenatal complications were found to be positively related to severity and chronicity of maternal psychiatric disturbance. However, the poor prenatal and obstetrical status of schizophrenic women in the Sameroff sample (10) was primarily due to chronic medication use, which was rated as an obstetrical complication in this study.

Similar to these findings for the prenatal period, data suggested that a positive association may exist between delivery complications and severity of maternal psychiatric disturbance (10). Data were contradictory (16), however, and the majority of studies did not indicate increased rates of delivery complications for schizophrenic women or women bearing the offspring of schizophrenic fathers compared with psychiatrically or socioeconomically matched controls (17). The extent to which these contradictory findings result from differences in the type and quality of prenatal care provided in different nations remains to be clarified.

Much of the data on the general status and neurointegrative functioning of the infant were also contradictory. Walker and Emory concluded that the bulk of the evidence on fetal/neonatal death and birth weight indicates no significant differences between children of schizophrenics and controls (17). However, McNeil and Kaij's finding that children of schizophrenics, compared with control children, were small for gestational age but not different in length, head circumference, or shoulder circumference warrants followup (18). Being small for gestational age or having a low ponderal index (weight-to-length ratio) may reflect intrauterine growth retardation, a factor that is associated with increased morbidity and, when extreme, has been linked with later learning and attentional problems. Findings of intrauterine growth retardation in children of schizophrenics would be particularly interesting given reports of erratic growth and deviations in musculoskeletal development during infancy for high-risk children (9, 19).

Results concerning the neurological and motor functioning of infants of schizophrenics were contradictory as well. Ehrlenmeyer-Kimling and Cornblatt (20) and Walker and Emory (17) concluded that the evidence was about evenly split concerning the presence or absence of abnormalities in neuromotor functioning in infants of schizophrenics. It is interesting to note, however, that whereas neurological abnormalities in most neonates tend to gradually improve, trends observed in offspring of schizophrenics suggest more severe deficits that persist throughout the first year of life (17). High variable sensitivity to sensory stimulation and abnormal levels of excitability may also be characteristics of children of schizophrenics, although again the data were conflicting (10, 19, 21, 22).

As discussed earlier, only a subgroup of children of schizophrenics are expected to have the genetic liability for schizophrenia. Consequently, analyses of overall group differences between high- and low-risk children may obscure important findings. Analyses of individual differences within high-risk groups in the infancy literature have suggested that this may be the case. In 3 of the 23 studies we reviewed, subgroups of infants of schizophrenics who showed deviant developmental patterns were identified (23-25), and in two studies subgroups of high-risk infants who showed deviant development were most likely to develop schizophrenic disorders in adolescence and early adulthood (24, 25). However, the type of deviant development examined in these studies differed. Fish's (24) disturbed sample showed pandysmaturation or periods when gross motor, visual motor, and physical development were transiently disorganized. In contrast, preschizophrenics and preschizotypal infants in the Danish sample were described as passive, unenergetic, and having short attention spans (25).

Early Childhood (Ages 2 to 4)

Early childhood appears to represent a neglected age span in risk research: Only four studies offer data on this developmental period. The trends observed in early childhood parallel those found in infancy. Support for the notion of a neurointegrative deficit in children of schizophrenics is provided by Sameroff's (10) finding that at age 2 1/2, children of schizophrenics tended to be less reactive than controls, as assessed on the Bayley Infant Behavior Record. Low reactivity was also associated with parental psychiatric severity and chronicity, with the severely disturbed mothers having the least reactive toddlers. Hanson et al. (26) reported that compared with children of nonschizophrenic psychiatric controls, four-year-old children of schizophrenics tended to show poor gross and fine motor performance. This was also consistent with the patterns of abnormal neuromotor development observed in infants of schizophrenics (26).

Findings of peculiarities in social functioning that are specific to children of schizophrenics are sparse. Sameroff et al. found more parental reports of depression in children of schizophrenics than in children of controls with no illness (10). In addition,

Hanson et al. reported that children of schizophrenics were more often described as schizoid (that is, emotionally flat, withdrawn, distractable, passive, irritable, and negativistic) (26). A subgroup of children of schizophrenics (17 percent of the high-risk sample) were also identified who were characterized by a) schizoid behavioral features both at age 4 and age 7, b) poor motor functioning, and c) large intraindividual variability on cognitive test performance. Most of these children also had family histories loaded with schizophrenia. These findings on social behavior in high-risk children are somewhat suspect due to the large number of analyses conducted, the strong possibility of chance findings, and the optimizing statistical procedures used. Moreover, the differences between children of schizophrenics and controls pale when contrasted with the variability noted within the offspring of schizophrenics as a function of the severity of parent's disorder. Sameroff found that maternal reports of global child disturbance at 30 months were related to severity and chronicity of maternal psychiatric disturbance (10). The children of the more chronically and severely disturbed mothers showed less cooperation with the family, more fearfulness, more bizarre behavior, and more depression. In addition, it was the children of depressed mothers, not schizophrenic mothers, who appeared to show the greatest social dysfunction.

Middle Childhood (Ages 5 to 12)

In contrast to the relative dearth of information concerning the adjustment of children of schizophrenics during early childhood, at least 12 studies reported data on high-risk children during the elementary school years. Considerable information concerning neurointegrative functioning in children of schizophrenics at this age is currently available. Since reviews of these data are available elsewhere, we highlight only major findings (20, 27-29) here.

Support for the hypothesis of a neurointegrative deficit in high-risk children during middle childhood comes from three different types of studies: 1) studies of autonomic responsivity, 2) studies of neurological and motor functioning, and 3) studies of attention and information processing. Results of studies on autonomic responsivity (as measured by electrodermal response) provide the weakest evidence supporting the hypothesis of a neurointegrative deficit in children of schizophrenics. Since Mednick and Schulsinger's original report (30) that rapid recovery of the skin conductance response was associated with subsequent psychiatric breakdown in their Danish sample, additional analyses of these data suggested that this relationship is complicated by gender and parental separation effects (31). Moreover, several other groups of investigators failed to find an association between risk status and electrodermal activity (for example, 20).

In contrast, reports on neurological and motor functioning in the eight samples in which these areas were assessed consistently indicated some impairment in some high-risk children (12, 24, 32-34). Review of these studies reveals that impaired fine motor coordination is the single sign reported by all investigators. Several investigators also reported delays in motor development similar to those found in studies of infancy and early childhood (10). In addition, Marcus et al. reported (35) that five of six children in the NIMH Israeli high-risk sample (32), who in preliminary analyses showed evidence of "schizophrenia spectrum psychoses," at the five-year followup (between the ages of 12 and 20) showed earlier difficulties in neurological functioning. All of these children showed problems in motor coordination, (for example, finger opposition, bringing the finger to the nose, rapid manipulation of matchsticks, copying geometric figures) and sensory perceptual functioning (for example, form perception, auditory visual integration, tactile discrimination).

Current evidence thus suggests that neurological impairments are more common in children of schizophrenics than in normal controls and may be associated with the development of schizophrenia during adolescence. These impairments for the most part do not reflect disturbances in vegetative or passive neurological functions. Rather, deficits in children of schizophrenics emerged most frequently in tasks assessing fine motor coordination, rate of motor development, and sensory perceptual functioning. It has been speculated that this pattern of deficits could stem from disruption of the frontal and parietal tertiary association cortex (27).

Attention and information processing in children of schizophrenics during middle childhood was also found to be impaired. In three of the five studies on attention and information processing in high-risk children between ages 5 and 12, some impairment in children of schizophrenics was found (20, 27). On relatively simple tasks, children of schizophrenics tended to respond similarly to normals (34, 36-39). However, with one exception (41), children of schizophrenics tended to show impairment on more complex tasks that assess performance under stimulus overload conditions (38, 40, 42, 43). Recent results also suggest that these attentional impairments may be associated with specific electrophysiological patterns (that is, reduced amplitude in late positive components of event-related electroencephalogram potentials (44).

Attempts to identify subgroups of high-risk children with

attention/ information processing dysfunction have proved particularly fruitful. Three of the five projects examining attention and information processing in high-risk children during middle childhood identified a subgroup of children who showed impaired performance (40, 42, 45), suggesting that attentional deficits are characteristic of only a subset of high-risk children. Preliminary adjustment data emerging from the New York project further indicate that high-risk children who have been hospitalized and/or treated during adolescence for psychiatric disorders tended to have deviant performance on attentional tasks, poorer neuromotor performance, and lower IQ scores, with a larger verbal compared with performance IQ deficit than did the remaining high-risk children and children with depressed or normal parents. Path analyses suggested a model whereby the genetic vulnerability to schizophrenia is expressed primarily in neuromotor functioning, which then leads to attentional disturbance, which subsequently influences clinical adjustment (37).

Results of examinations of general intellectual functioning in middle childhood generally suggest that children of schizophrenics do not show clinically significant differences in IQ relative to controls. There is some evidence, however, of a slightly lower IQ in children of schizophrenics compared with controls (46-48). Three studies linking verbal IQ deficits to behavior disturbance are particularly noteworthy. Ehrlenmeyer-Kimling reported lower verbal IQ in high-risk children treated during adolescence (37). Fish reported a correlation between increases in schizotypal symptoms and a drop in scores on the Comprehension subtest of the Verbal Scale of the Wechsler Intelligence Scale for Children--Revised between ages 10 and 15 (24). Reider and Nichols found depressed performance on the Comprehension subtest in a subset of high-risk boys who also showed neurological signs and behavioral indices of hyperactivity, impulsivity, short attention span, and emotional lability (12). These data suggest that specific verbal intellectual functions may be more sensitive to developing schizophrenic dysfunction than more global summary scores.

Consistent with the data from earlier age periods, data on middle childhood indicate that some children of schizophrenic parents tend to show disturbed social functioning compared with children of normal controls. However, impaired social role functioning appears to have been related to the severity of parental disturbance rather than to parental schizophrenia. The degree of social dysfunction found in children of schizophrenics is also relatively minimal in comparison to the degree of social dysfunction found in groups of clinically disturbed children (40, 49). No specific deficit in social functioning has been identified exclusively in children of schizophrenics. Rather, like many other child clinical and risk groups, some children of schizophrenics have been found to be negatively evaluated by their peers; rated as aggressive and disruptive by peers and teachers; rated as low in social and cognitive competence by peers and teachers; and described as emotionally flat, withdrawn, distractable, passive, irritable, negativistic, hyperactive, emotionally labile, and immature (6, 12, 26, 40, 49-52). It should be noted however, that these social deficits were not found in all children in all high-risk samples.

Adolescence

Although high-risk-research investigators generally plan to follow children through adolescence, only 3 of the 23 studies being reviewed began with adolescents. Five additional projects either included young adolescents within a mostly preadolescent sample or followed an initially younger sample into adolescence. Several findings emerged on the adolescent adjustment of children at risk for schizophrenia. Consistent with findings for earlier developmental phases, a number of signs of neurointegrative deficits were found. In the one examination of neurointegrative functioning in adolescent children of schizophrenics (35), deficits were found in motor coordination, balance, and sensory perceptual signs. A disproportionate number of children of schizophrenic parents showed neurological dysfunction on from three to five of the six possible neurological areas evaluated. As noted earlier, although only very early data are currently available, known adolescent schizophrenia spectrum breakdowns tended to occur in children with signs of neuromotor dysfunction during middle childhood, adolescence, or both periods.

Data on attention and information processing in adolescent children of schizophrenics also points to a neurointegrative deficit in high-risk children. Asarnow et al. (52) found that when compared with foster and community controls, biological children of schizophrenics who had been placed in foster homes performed more poorly on a series of complex attention-demanding tasks. A subgroup of high-risk children were identified who both manifested impairment on a number of tasks and showed evidence of clinical difficulties. These children tended to report high scores on the Schizophrenic and Psychopathic Deviate scales of the Minnesota Multiphasic Personality Inventory, micropsychotic experiences, more problems with social isolation, and greater difficulty in meeting the student role (53). The reevaluation of subjects at adolescence in the New York Project generally yielded comparable findings (37). Although these investigators have not yet reported the relationships among adolescent clinical, attentional, and neuromotor functioning, the attentional and neuromotor measures obtained during middle childhood were related to adolescent clinical status.

Consistent with the notion that increasing psychopathology is associated with a decline in IQ, data on general intellectual functioning showed somewhat greater evidence of impairment in high-risk children as they enter adolescence and approach the high-risk period for schizophrenia. Striking evidence of this sort is provided by Fish's (54) description of Edwin, whose Verbal and Performance IQs declined steadily from 10 to 15 years of age. Other evidence supporting this notion is provided by Worland's (55) report of significantly lower IQ scores for children of schizophrenic and manic-depressive parents compared with children of nonpsychotic parents during adolescence, but not during middle childhood. Interestingly, children of schizophrenics had the lowest correlations between IQ scores during these two age periods, suggesting less continuity and perhaps some disruption in intellectual functioning for the high-risk adolescents. Reports from the Danish (30) and New York (56) studies also suggest somewhat lower intellectual functioning in adolescents at risk for schizophrenia. Signs of more general cognitive disturbance were also reported in high-risk adolescents (48) as well as in high-risk children who later developed schizophrenia spectrum disorders (25).

Results concerning impaired social functioning in high-risk adolescents are remarkably consistent. Studies that included or started with adolescent samples without exception showed some evidence of social dysfunction in high-risk samples. Similar to findings during middle childhood, many of the deviant social patterns observed in adolescents at risk for schizophrenia are also found in other clinical and risk populations (57). Recent outcome data from the Danish project (58), however, suggest that two areas of social impairment characterizing adolescent risk samples merit particular attention. In particular, teachers' reports of poor affective control (easily upset, affect persists when excited, disturbs class by unusual behavior, presents disciplinary problems) and difficulty making friends were found to discriminate adolescent children of schizophrenics who had schizophrenic episodes during late adolescence or early adulthood from high-risk children with healthy outcomes. Poor affective control in school was correlated with clinical ratings of formal cognitive disturbance, whereas difficulty making friends was related to clinical ratings of poor emotional rapport. These correlations imply that poor affective control and poor interpersonal relationships may comprise two major dimensions of prepsychotic social behavior, each of which is correlated with a different but crucial diagnostic symptom of schizophrenia.

In sum, in the 23 projects in which the offspring of schizophrenics were studied, three attributes appeared repeatedly: 1) a difficult pregnancy and delivery, 2) signs of neuropsychological and attentional deficits that persist beyond infancy, and 3) disturbances in social behavior best characterized as poor affective control that is linked to poor peer relationships. These findings require that we view the results of these diverse studies at a high level of conceptual abstraction since the measures used at different age levels or in different studies are in the same behavioral domain (measures of attention) even if the specific measures often varied in a number of ways. Thus credibility of these findings depends on whether one agrees or disagrees with how we have assigned specific measures to these conceptual domains of behavior. Also, we must emphasize that the attributes identified are true not for all offspring of schizophrenic parents but only a subset of these youngsters. However, it is encouraging that these studies, in which cohorts have been followed into the early stages of the high-risk period of schizophrenia, have found that members of that subset are at higher risk for severe psychopathology or schizophrenia.

What about the third question that high-risk research is designed to answer? Do these attributes identify a person at risk specifically for schizophrenia, or do they simply identify one at risk for severe psychopathology? We are limited in our ability to determine whether the attributes summarized are vulnerability markers specific to schizophrenia or are general precursors of adult psychopathology. One way to examine this issue is to see whether the attributes are found only in offspring of schizophrenics and not in offspring of parents who have other psychiatric conditions. Reliability of such a comparison is grounded on the results of family genetic studies of schizophrenic cohorts, which support the notion of specificity of transmission across generations. Thus, if something is a vulnerability marker for schizophrenia it should appear only in the offspring of schizophrenics. A major difficulty in evaluating the specificity of the attributes found in this review of the 23 studies is that not all of the studies used three-group design (that is, including a nonschizophrenic, nonpsychiatric comparison group). When the three-group design was used, the findings concerning specificity were not overwhelming. However, the best evidence for specificity of attributes comes from the Israeli high-risk study (Dr. Allen Mirsky, personal communication, April 1985), in which evidence for cognitive and attentional deficits was most common in the offspring of schizophrenics. Thus, if there is any evidence for specificity, it is in this behavioral domain.

The reader may wonder why the issue of specificity of a risk marker is so important for identifying individuals likely to profit from a preventive intervention program. If one wishes to use a risk marker within a cohort with schizophrenic parentage, the risk marker need not be highly specific because it may serve to identify that subset of individuals already at risk by virtue of parental mental illness. The specificity comes from the close statistical correspondence between the form of parental and offspring mental disorder. Within that context, nonspecific vulnerability markers can be very valuable. If, however, one wishes to screen large unselected populations to find groups at risk for schizophrenia, the lack of vulnerability markers specific to that disorder poses real problems. Since, as we indicated previously, only 10 percent of schizophrenic persons have the risk marker of parental mental illness, the identification of specific vulnerability markers (or clusters of them) would greatly expand our capability to mount effective preventive intervention programs.

The fourth and final issue that high-risk research is designed to study is whether there are specific attributes of the family environment that predispose one to schizophrenia and may identify high-risk family units. There is frequent mention in the high-risk literature of parent-child disturbances. Collectively, these data on early infant and mother behavior point to abnormal patterns of mother-infant interaction between some schizophrenics and their children from the earliest stages of life. Many of these differences appear to be associated with general risk factors such as severity of maternal disturbance and socioeconomic status. Although it is difficult and perhaps relatively unimportant to evaluate the predominant directionality of effects (mother to infant versus infant to mother), it is likely that reciprocal influences begin at birth and perhaps prenatally. High rates of parental stress and risk-increasing behavior in schizophrenic women may lead to increased prenatal and delivery complications that may in turn create or exacerbate subtle neurointegrative abnormalities in the child. Similarly, an infant who has suffered erratic intrauterine growth may enter the world with neurointegrative deficits and a difficult temperament. When that child is given to a stressed and psychiatrically disturbed mother who provides her child with a negative affective environment in which to grow, the child may develop an increasingly difficult temperament and show nonoptimal cognitive, emotional, and social growth.

Studies of family functioning in the middle childhood period yielded few family variables specific to families of schizophrenics.

Consistent with findings from families with children in earlier age periods, families of schizophrenics containing 6- to 12-year-old children were characterized by a number of negative attributes. However these negative attributes were also characteristic of families of other types of psychiatric patients. Compared with normal families, families containing schizophrenic patients were characterized by poor marital adjustment, low levels of solidarity, poor children's relationships, poor household facilities, and high rates of financial problems (49). In addition, as in the early childhood period, families with psychotic (including but not exclusively schizophrenic) as opposed to nonpsychotic parents were found to show low rates of interaction, low family warmth, low rates of parental behavior requests, and high rates of sibling rivalry (59, 60, and Worland et al.'s [1983] unpublished manuscript). Parents with the most severe dysfunction tended to show the least interaction and warmth in their family interactions. In contrast, children of normal parents tended to perceive their parents as having more positive feelings toward them than their parents actually expressed toward them on the Family Relations Test. Children of psychotic parents often did not show this tendency toward a positively skewed affect (Worland et al. [1984] unpublished manuscript). This could be related to the lack of warmth in families with psychotic and severely disturbed parents.

In one study, family interaction patterns were examined in a sample of moderately disturbed teenagers, some of whom were hypothesized to be at risk for schizophrenia (61, 62). Two major dimensions of parental behavior were examined. One was communication deviance, which measures the parent's inability to maintain a shared focus of attention during transactions with others. The other was an affective component of parental behavior consisting of negative affective style, which reflects behavior in directly observed family interaction (63), and expressed emotion, which reflects attitudes towards another family member expressed during an interview (64). This study differed from others in that it was not restricted to offspring of schizophrenic parents and the results may be generalizable to larger populations. These adolescents were then followed for 15 years and the incidence of schizophrenia-spectrum disorders observed. If we examine the incidence of schizophrenia-spectrum disorders in any offspring in the family (see Figure 1) we can see that in families with high levels of communication deviance, the rate of subsequent schizophrenia-spectrum disorders was very high, hovering around 45 percent for a narrow definition of the extended schizophrenia spectrum and even higher if such conditions as schizoid and borderline personality disorder were included. Further, it was found

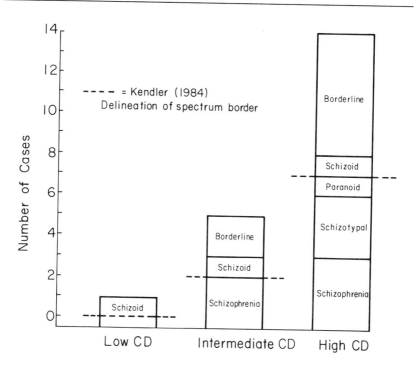

Figure 1. Number of cases (index or sibling as most severe) diagnosed schizophrenia spectrum at follow-up (*N* = 12), intermediate (*N* = 20), or high (*N* = 19) parental communication deviance (CD) level for narrow and spectrum categories (Kendler).

that all cases of schizophrenia had families characterized by high communication deviance and negative affective style and high expressed emotion.

Some degree of indirect confirmation for family patterns as risk markers comes from the Finnish Adoption Study (65) of Tienari, who found that the only cases of schizophrenia in the adopted-away offspring of schizophrenic parents occurred in adoptive families rated as disturbed. Thus there is some presumptive evidence that measures such as communication deviance, affective style, and expressed emotion, in combination, can identify family units at risk for schizophrenia or related disorders in one or more offspring.

OVERVIEW AND IMPLICATIONS FOR PREVENTION

The potential pathways to schizophrenia are diagrammed in Figure 2 to assist the reader in placing the findings reviewed in this

chapter in longitudinal perspective. The diagram should help identify possible strategies for future prevention research. Three areas
appear worthy of further prevention-oriented research. The first is
based on the prenatal-early infancy findings that link psychiatric
disturbance of the mother, pregnancy and birth complications,
early signs of neurointegrative deficit and disturbed parent-child
relationships during infancy. Thus one focus of prevention research could be to alter the course of pregnancies in mothers who
have a history of schizophrenia, thereby lessening the likelihood of
pregnancy and birth complications, and to attempt during the
postnatal period to stimulate a more favorable parent-child interaction. We could then examine whether these interventions
reduce the incidence of neuropsychological anomalies in the offspring of schizophrenic parents. Further follow-ups could indicate
whether subsequent neurological and attentional capabilities have
thereby been normalized.

The second area worthy of prevention research is indicated by
the recurrent evidence that children at risk demonstrate in middle
childhood notable deficits in attentional-information processing
tasks. We should attempt some interventions with these children to
determine if the deficits are modifiable or correctable. Given the
impressive evidence of the continuity and magnification of these
cognitive deficits with age, any improvement in these capabilities
could very well serve a protective function in reducing the probability of a subsequent schizophrenic episode.

Third, it appears that it may be possible to identify high-risk
family units among those seeking help for their youngsters, using
measures of communication deviance, affective style, and expressed emotion. Targeted intervention programs could be designed to evaluate the modifiability of these parental attributes and
the subsequent course of the offspring's psychiatric and social
functioning.

Prevention of the Reoccurrence of Schizophrenia

It should be obvious that the preventive efforts outlined in this
chapter begin with some individual or family unit showing signs
of distress or deficit states. Thus, the focus of preventive intervention is to alter the life course of persons at risk who have already deviated from a healthy trajectory. But preventive efforts
need not be confined to this type of life-course modification. For
no one is at more risk for schizophrenia than someone who has
had an initial episode of a schizophrenic disorder. Thus, it could
be argued that we need to expand our prevention efforts to this
population as well. Anything that can be done to prevent another

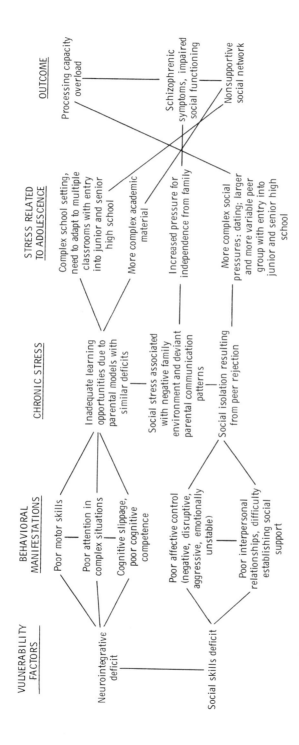

Figure 2. A tentative model for the development of schizophrenia that integrates the results of data from 23 high-risk studies.

episode of schizophrenia in a young person in particular can have a major impact on that person's life course. Fortunately, there are a number of favorable signs that affected individuals can benefit from programs that combine maintenance pharmacotherapy with programs of family support and intervention. A review of the programs tested so far indicated positive short-term results (66). Better preventive intervention programs must be designed for young, early-onset schizophrenic patients and their families that can go beyond short-term prevention of relapse. More research and more dissemination of these programs to clinical practitioners is needed to prevent the deadly cycle of repeated episodes of this dread disorder.

REFERENCES

1. Goldstein MJ (Editor): Preventive Intervention in Schizophrenia: Are We Ready? (DHHS Publication No. ADM 82-111). Washington, DC, U.S. Government Printing Office, 1982
2. Bloom BL, Hodges WF, Kern MK, et al: A preventive intervention program for the newly separated: final evaluations. Am J Orthopsychiatry 55:9-26, 1985
3. Cowen EL: Choices and alternatives for primary prevention in mental health research, in Preventive Interventions in Schizophrenia: Are We Ready? (DHHS Publication No. ADM 178-191). Edited by Goldstein MJ. Washington, DC, U.S. Government Printing Office, 1982
4. Garmezy N, Streitman S: Children at risk: the search for antecedents of schizophrenia. I. Conceptual models and research methods. Schizophr Bull 1:14-90 1974
5. Garmezy N: Children at risk: the search for the antecedents of schizophrenia. II. Ongoing research programs, issues and, intervention. Schizophr Bull 9:55-125, 1974
6. Asarnow JR, Goldstein MJ: Schizophrenia during adolescence and early adulthood: a developmental perspective on risk research. Clinical Psychology Review, in press
7. McNeil TF, Kaij L, Malmquist-Larsson A: Pregnant women with nonorganic psychosis: life situation and experience of pregnancy. Acta Psychiatr Scand 68:445-457, 1983
8. Wrede G: Finnish children with schizophrenic mothers: a prospective risk group study, in Children at Risk for Schizophrenia: A Longitudinal Perspective. Edited by Watt N, Anthony EJ, Wynne L, et al. New York, Cambridge University Press, 1984
9. Ragins N, Schachter J, Elmer E: Infants and children at risk

for schizophrenia. J Child Psychiatry 14:150-177, 1975

10. Sameroff AJ, Seifer R, Zax M: Early development of children at risk for emotional disorder. Monographs of the Society for Research in Child Development 47:Serial 199, 1982

11. Mednick S, Mura E, Schulsinger F, et al: Perinatal conditions and infant development in children with schizophrenic parents. Soc Biol 18:103-113, 1971

12. Rieder R, Nichols P: Offspring of schizophrenics. III. Arch Gen Psychiatry 36:665-674, 1979

13. Rieder R, Rosenthal D, Wender P, et al: The offspring of schizophrenics: fetal and neonatal deaths. Arch Gen Psychiatry 32:200-211, 1975

14. Schachter J, Kerr J, Lachin J, et al: Newborn offspring of mentally disordered women. Am J Orthopsychiatry 47:218-230, 1977

15. Zax M, Sameroff A, Babigian H: Birth outcomes in the offspring of mentally disordered women. Am J Orthopsychiatry 47:218-230, 1977

16. McNeil T, Kaij L: Obstetric complications and physical size of offspring of schizophrenic, schizophrenic-like, and control mothers. Br J Psychiatry 123:341-348, 1973

17. Walker E, Emory E: Infants at risk for psychopathology: offspring of schizophrenic parents. Child Dev 54:1269-1285, 1983

18. McNeil TF, Kaij L, Malmquist-Larsson A, et al: Offspring of women with nonorganic psychoses. Development of a longitudinal study of children at high risk. Acta Psychiatr Scand 68:234-250, 1983

19. Fish B: Neurobiologic antecedents of schizophrenia in children: evidence for an inherited, congenital neurointegrative defect. Arch Gen Psychiatry 34:1297-1313, 1977

20. Ehrlenmeyer-Kimling L, Cornblatt B: Biobehavioral risk factors in schizophrenia parents. J Autism Dev Disord 14:357-374, 1984

21. Fish B: Biologic antecedents of psychosis in children, in Biology of the Major Psychoses. Edited by Freedman D. New York, Raven Press, 1975

22. McNeil TF, Kaij L: Offspring of women with nonorganic psychoses: progress report, in Children at Risk for Schizophrenia: A Longitudinal Prospective. Edited by Watt N, Anthony EJ, Wynne L, et al. New York, Cambridge University Press, 1984

23. Marcus J, Auerbach J, Wilkinson L, et al: Infants at risk for schizophrenia. Arch Gen Psychiatry 38:703-713, 1981

24. Fish B: Antecedents of an "acute" schizophrenic break. J Am Acad Child Psychiatry, in press

25. Parnas J, Schulsinger F, Teasdale T, et al: Perinatal complications and clinical outcome within the schizophrenia spectrum. Br J Psychiatry 140:421-424, 1982

26. Hanson D, Gottesman I, Heston L: Some possible childhood indicators of adult schizophrenia inferred from children of schizophrenics. Br J Psychiatry 129:142-154, 1976

27. Asarnow JR: Children with peer adjustment problem: sequential and nonsequential analyses of school behaviors. J Consult Clin Psychol 51:709-717, 1983

28. Nuechterlein KH, Phipps-Yonas S, Driscoll R, et al: Attential functioning among children vulnerable to adult schizophrenia, in Children at Risk for Schizophrenia: A Longitudinal Prospective.Edited by Watt N, Anthony EJ, Wynne L, et al. New York, Cambridge University Press, 1982

29. Nuechterlein N, Dawson ME: Information processing and attentional functioning in the developmental course of schizophrenic disorders. Schizophr Bull 10:160-203, 1984

30. Mednick S, Schulsinger F: Some premorbid characteristics related to breakdown in children with schizophrenic mothers, in The Transmission of Schizophrenia. Edited by Rosenthal D, Kety S. New York, Pergamon, 1968

31. Mednick SA, Schulsinger F, Teasdale TW, et al: Schizophrenia in high-risk children: sex differences in predisposing factors, in Cognitive Defects in the Development of Mental Illness. Edited by Serban G. New York, Brunner/Mazel, 1978

32. Rosenthal D: A program of research on heredity in schizophrenia. Behav Sci 16:191-201, 1971

33. Marcuse Y, Cornblatt B: Children at high risk for schizophrenia: predictions from infancy to childhood functioning, in Life Span Research on the Prediction of Psychopathology. Edited by Ehrlenmeyer-Kimling L, Miller N. New Jersey, Erlbaum, in press

34. Orvaschel H, Mednick S, Schulsinger F, et al: The children of psychiatrically disturbed parents. Arch Gen Psychiatry 36:691-695, 1979

35. Marcus J, Hans SL, Lewow E, et al: Neurological findings in the offspring of schizophrenics: childhood assessment and five-year following. Schizophr Bull 11:85-100, 1985

36. Cohler BJ, Grunebaum HU, Weiss JL, et al: Disturbances of attention among schizophrenic, depressed and well mothers and their children. J Child Psychol Psychiatry 18:115-135, 1971

37. Ehrlenmeyer-Kimling L, Cornblatt B, Friedman D, et al: Neurological, electrophysiological and attentional deviations in children at risk for schizophrenia, in Schizophrenia as a Brain Disease. Edited by Henn FA, Nasrallah HA.New York, Oxford

University Press, 1982

38. Ehrlenmeyer-Kimling L, Cornblatt B, Golden R: Early indicators of vulnerability to schizophrenia in children at high genetic risk, in Childhood Psychopathology and Development. Edited by Guze SB, Earls FJ, Barrett JE. New York, Raven Press, 1983

39. Herman J, Mirsky AF, Ricks NL, et al: Behavioral and electrographic measures of attention in children at risk for schizophrenia. J Abnorm Psychol 86:27-33, 1977

40. Nuechterlein KH: Signal detection in vigilance tasks and behavioral attributes among offspring of schizophrenic mothers and among hyperactive children. J Abnorm Psychol 92:4-28, 1983

41. Harvey P, Weintraub S, Neale J: Span of apprehension deficits in children vulnerable to psychopathology: a failure to replicate. J Abnorm Psychol 94:410-413, 1985

42. Cornblatt B, Ehrlenmeyer-Kimling L: Early attentional predictors of adolescent behavioral disturbances in children at risk for schizophrenia, in Children at Risk for Schizophrenia: A Longitudinal Perspective. Edited by Watt N, Anthony EJ, Wynne L, et al. New York, Cambridge University Press, 1984

43. Rutschmann J, Cornblatt B, Ehrlenmeyer-Kimling L: Sustained attention in children at risk for schizophrenia: report on a continuous performance test. Arch Gen Psychiatry 34:571-575, 1977

44. Friedman D, Vaughan H, Ehrlenmyer-Kimling L: Cognitive brain potentials in children at risk for schizophrenia: preliminary findings. Schizophr Bull 8:514-531, 1982

45. Winters KC, Stone AA, Weintraub S, et al: Cognitive and attentional deficits in children vulnerable to psychopathology. J Abnorm Child Psychol 9:435-453, 1981

46. Gruzelier J, Mednick S, Schulsinger F: Lateralized impairments in the WISC profiles of children at genetic risk for psychopathology, in Hemisphere Asymmetries of Function in Psychopathology. Edited by Gruzelier J, Flor-Henry P. Amsterdam, Elsevier/North Holland, 1979

47. Watt NF, Fryer JH, Lewine RJ, et al: Toward longitudinal conceptions of psychiatric disorder, in Progress in Experimental Personality Research. Edited by Maher BA. New York, Academic Press, 1979

48. Weintraub S, Neale J: The Stony Brook high-risk project, in Children at Risk for Schizophrenia: A Longitudinal Perspective. Edited by Watt N, Anthony EJ, Wynne LC, et al. New York, Cambridge University Press, 1984

49. Rolf JE: The academic and social competence of children vul-

nerable to schizophrenia and other behavior pathologies. J Abnorm Psychol 80:225-243, 1972

50. Fisher L, Harder D, Kokes R, et al: School functioning of children at risk for behavioral pathology, in Parental Pathology, Family Interaction and the Competence of the Child in School. Edited by Baldwin A, Cole R, Baldwin C. Monographs of the Society for Research in Child Development 47:12-16, 1982

51. Watt NF: Patterns of childhood social development in adult schizophrenics. Arch Gen Psychiatry 35:160-165, 1978

52. Asarnow R, Steffy R, MacCrimmon D, et al: An attentional assessment of foster children at risk for schizophrenia. J Abnorm Psychol 86:267-275, 1977

53. MacCrimmon DJ, Cleghorn JM, Asarnow RF, et al: Children at risk for schizophrenia. Arch Gen Psychiatry 37:671-674, 1980

54. Fish B:Characteristics and sequelae of the neurointegrative disorder in infants at risk for schizophrenia, in Children at Risk for Schizophrenia: A Longitudinal Perspective. Edited by Watt N, Anthony EJ, Wynne L, et al. New York, Cambridge University Press, 1984

55. Worland J, Edenhart-Pepe R, Weeks DG, et al: Cognitive evaluation of children at risk: IQ, differentiation, and egocentricity, in Children at Risk for Schizophrenia: A Longitudinal Perspective. Edited by Watt NF, Anthony EJ, Wynne LC, et al. New York, Cambridge University Press, 1984

56. Watt N, Grubb T, Ehrlenmeyer-Kimling L: Social, emotional, intellectual behavior at school among children at high risk for schizophrenia. J Consult Clin Psychol 50:171-181, 1982

57. Asarnow JR: The Waterloo studies of interpersonal competence, in Children at Risk for Schizophrenia: A Longitudinal Perspective. Edited by Watt N, Anthony EJ, Wynne L, et al. New York, Cambridge University Press, 1984

58. Parnas J, Schulsinger F, Schulsinger H, et al: Behavioral precursors of schizophrenia spectrum. Arch Gen Psychiatry 39:658-664, 1982

59. Baldwin AL, Cole RE, Baldwin CP, et al: The role of family interaction in mediating the effect of parental pathology upon the school functioning of the child. Monographs of the Society for Research in Child Development 47:1-11, 1982

60. Baldwin AL, Baldwin CP, Cole RE: Family freeplay interaction: settings and methods. Monographs for the Society for Research in Child Development 47:72-80, 1982

61. Goldstein MJ, Rodnick EH, Jones JE, et al: Familial precursors of schizophrenia spectrum disorders, in The Nature of

Schizophrenia. Edited by Wynne LC, Cromwell RL, Matthysse S. New York, Wiley, 1978

62. Goldstein MJ: Family factors that antedate the onset of schizophrenia and related disorders: the results of a fifteen year prospective longitudinal study. Acta Psychiatr Scand 71:7-18, 1985

63. Doane JA, West KL, Goldstein MJ: Parental communication deviance and affective style: predictors of subsequent spectrum disorders in vulnerable adolescents. Arch Gen Psychiatry 38:679-685 1981

64. Vaughn CE, Leff JP: The influence of family and social factors on the course of psychiatric illness. Br J Psychiatry 129:125-137, 1976

65. Tienari P, Sorri A, Naarala M, et al: The Finnish adoptive family study: adopted-away offspring of schizophrenic mothers, in Psychosocial Intervention in Schizophrenia. Edited by Stierlin H, Wynne LC, Wirsching M. Berlin, Springer-Verlag, 1983

66. Goldstein MJ (Editor): New Directions for Mental Health Services: New Developments in Interventions With Families of Schizophrenics. San Francisco, Jossey-Bass, 1981

6

Primary Prevention of
Alcohol and Substance Abuse

Richard J. Frances, M.D.

John E. Franklin, M.D.

6

Primary Prevention of
Alcohol and Substance Abuse

Increased study of risk factors in alcoholism and substance abuse during the past decade has been accompanied by a search for a way to prevent addictive illnesses. Considering that approximately one out of every four or five sons of alcoholics becomes alcoholic and that a family history of alcoholism increases the risk in both sexes four or five times, the need for primary prevention is crucial (1).

The biopsychosocial model of the illness suggests various approaches to prevention. For example, the important etiological role of hereditary and familial factors in either adding to vulnerability or protecting against the problem raises the possibility of identifying high-risk populations, searching for biological markers, and developing strategies for prevention in children of alcoholics. Effects of social planning, law enforcement, and public education have also received attention. The public has become increasingly interested and better informed about addictions in recent years. Betty Ford, Rosalynn Carter, and Nancy Reagan have discussed addictions and emotional problems and thus contributed to public education. The current generation of Americans pursues health and physical fitness while struggling with choices about alcohol and drugs.

In this chapter, recent developments in the field of primary prevention of alcohol and substance abuse are presented, including, identifying high-risk populations, increasing public education, limiting the availability of substances, and designing social policies that will lead to prevention. In addition, a discussion of the psychiatrist's role in early detection, careful diagnosis, and treatment as well as suggestions to help families break the endless cycle of addictions are presented.

THE ROLE OF PREVENTION

The greatest advances in medicine have been effected by development of means to prevent illnesses. In order for this to be accomplished, the illness needs to be well understood in terms of its description, etiology, pathogenesis, course, and epidemiology. The prevention of infectious disease by vaccination and parasitic disease by improved sanitary and public health measures are examples of successful primary prevention programs. In alcoholism and substance dependency, we are still at the stage in which diagnosis is the product of a committee, etiology is unknown, longitudinal data are scanty, and the effects of social policy are not well studied. Prohibition was a dramatic prevention attempt that failed because of the lack of understanding of the complexities involved. The vast cost of the problem requires greater investment in research to develop a better understanding of the illness, its prevention, and its treatment than is currently undertaken. At the same time, we must find ways to effectively apply current knowledge of prevention and treatment to make choices about the best way to invest limited resources.

MAGNITUDE OF THE PROBLEM

Efforts are currently underway to quantify the extent of psychiatric illnesses in the general population. This knowledge is important to justify allocation of funds for primary prevention. Robbins et al. recently reported on the lifetime prevalence rates for psychiatric disorders in a large ongoing National Institute of Mental Health (NIMH) epidemiological study (2). Substance abuse disorders rank first among 15 *DSM-III* diagnoses, with an average of 13.3 percent of the general population having a lifetime prevalence of alcohol abuse or dependence and 5.6 percent prevalence of drug abuse or dependence across three catchment areas. Myers et al., looking at six-month prevalence rates in the general population, reported a five percent rate of alcohol abuse or dependence and a two percent rate of drug abuse or dependence (3). In a recent University of Michigan study of 17,000 high school seniors, 29 percent of the students said they had used alcohol or drugs in the month before the survey, and 62 percent said they had tried an illegal substance at least once in their lifetime (4). In a 1983 survey among New York high school students, 67 percent reported having had past involvement with illegal or nonmedical substance use, and one-third reported having tried illegal drugs by the time they were in seventh grade (5).

The 1-800-COCAINE hotline received over one million calls in its first two years of operation, and this has led to a greater public awareness of the growing dangers of a cocaine epidemic (6, 7). While recent evidence points to a leveling off or decline of drug use among adolescents, perhaps as a result of preventive efforts, this does not include cocaine use, which has been dangerously on the rise (7, 8). Americans consume an estimated 50 metric tons of cocaine annually, at a cost of 39 billion dollars. Cocaine is often used with other drugs such as opiates, barbiturates, and alcohol to take the "edge off" the effects of cocaine. In Latin American countries, where cocaine is widely available as a paste, use is epidemic and constitutes a major public health problem. A current decline in the cost of cocaine presents a major threat to American youth (7).

Alcoholism is the third largest health problem in the United States, directly affecting 14 million people (9). In 1981, 43 percent of street and highway deaths involved alcohol. Niven estimated the deletethisline

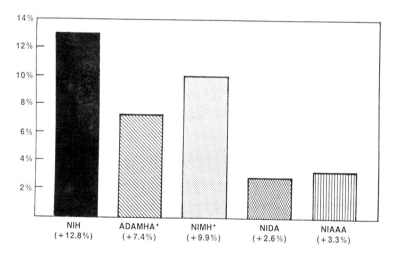

Figure 1. 1985 appropriation: percentage of increase over President's request. NIH = National Institutes of Health; ADAMHA = Alcohol, Drug Abuse, and Mental Health Administration; NIMH = National Institute of Mental Health; NIDA = National Institute on Drug Abuse; NIAAA = National Institute on Alcohol Abuse and Alcoholism. *Excludes block grant, Community Support Program, and clinical training.

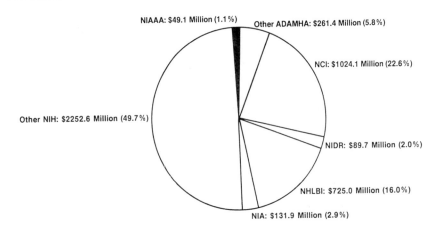

Figure 2. Research distribution on resources for the institutes of the Alcohol, Drug Abuse, and Mental Health Administration (ADAMHA) and the National Institutes of Health (NIH) for Fiscal Year 1985. NIAAA = National Institute on Alcohol Abuse and Alcoholism; NCI = National Cancer Institute; NIDR = National Institute of Dental Research; NHLBI = National Heart, Lung, and Blood Institute; NIA = National Institute on Aging.

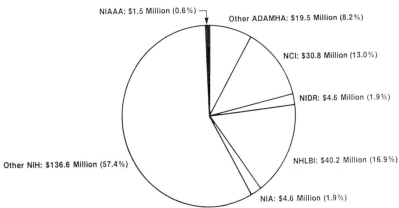

Figure 3. Research training distribution of resources for the institutes of the Alcohol, Drug Abuse, and Mental Health Administration (ADAMHA) and the National Institutes of Health (NIH) for Fiscal Year 1985. NIAAA = National Institute on Alcohol Abuse and Alcoholism; NCI = National Cancer Institute; NIDR = National Institute of Dental Research; NHLBI = National Heart, Lung, and Blood Institute; NIA = National Institute on Aging.

cost to society of alcoholism to be approximately 116 billion dollars annually (10).

Although awareness of the problem has increased, the National Institute of Alcohol Abuse and Alcoholism (NIAAA) and the National Institute on Drug Abuse have not received increases in research funding on a par with funds allocated to other National Institutes of Health programs, including the Alcohol, Drug Abuse, and Mental Health Administration (ADAMHA) and the National Institute of Mental Health (Figure 1). The NIAAA receives 1.1 percent of monies spent at national institutes, down from 1.3 percent in 1983 (Figure 2). In compliance with President Reagan's request for budget cutbacks, research grants will be funded at only 90 percent of their approved level. Research training in alcoholism was funded at 1.5 million in 1985, which is below the corrected inflation dollar amount for 1978 and is less than half the relative percentage of extramural research for ADAMHA.

Only 0.6 percent of all national training funds support alcoholism research, despite the fact that alcoholism is a major public health problem and that an increase in funding is essential if bright researchers are to be recruited to work on the problem (Figure 3). Indeed, the Institute of Medicine has recommended more than doubling the NIAAA's research budget (Figure 4).

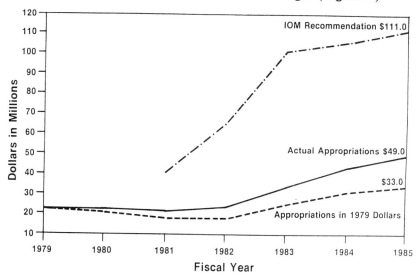

Figure 4. National Institute on Alcohol Abuse and Alcoholism research appropriations compared with Institute of Medicine recommendation. Recommendation was for a 50 percent increase for three years, with only inflation adjustments thereafter.

EDUCATIONAL PROGRAMS

In taking a biopsychosocial approach to studying a disease, one considers it from a host agent and environment viewpoint. Most primary prevention efforts have focused on school- and work-based alcohol education programs, mass media campaigns, and limitation of the availability of the agent. Educational programs have been developed for students, parents, and employees. School-based education efforts have significantly increased knowledge regarding alcohol and substance abuse. Although people are more aware of the problems caused by addiction, less dramatic changes in attitudes toward alcohol have resulted. Changes in drinking behavior have generally been modest or difficult to demonstrate (11).

Goodstadt and Sheppard studied strategies for improving cognitive, decision-making, and value clarification abilities among children regarding drugs (12). In their study, cognitive interventions increased knowledge but produced no result in attitude or behavioral change. Decision-making techniques were effective when affectual components were included in the design, but value clarification techniques were not useful. Prior learning styles, expectations, differing abilities, and backgrounds must be taken into account when devising a school based program.

Adolescents often experience pleasurable effects from alcohol and drug experimentation. For children of alcoholics and other high-risk groups a total abstinence strategy makes good sense. However, use of this approach with other adolescents may undermine a program's credibility, and thus its effectiveness, because alcohol is a ubiquitous symbolic social lubricator in American society. Coming to personal terms with alcohol and substance abuse may represent a developmental task for some teenagers. Programs that are broadly conceived and touch upon myths about alcohol, alcohol advertisement, causes of alcoholism, and the effects of alcohol on one's satisfaction with life are most successful.

Prevention programs based on social learning theory emphasize teaching young people how to refuse drugs. Such programs provide information about the hazards of drugs, peer pressure, and one's specific behavioral repertoire for saying no. The underlying assumption is that rehearsal of various rejecting responses will increase the likelihood they will be used in appropriate situations. Johnson et al. described one such program, "Project Smart," for sixth to ninth graders that utilized peer leaders to enhance social resistance skills and improve self-management (13). Techniques included discussion, demonstration, and role playing. A current television commercial reinforces the simple message of "Project Smart": The commercial is "Just Say No."

Factors identified with adolescent alcohol abuse include peer pressure, parental modeling, a desire to obtain adult status, curiosity, low self-esteem, and unstable families. Peer pressure is paramount. Greater adolescent drug use is associated with an increased sense of autonomy and independence from parents and unconventionality. Drugs may be used to solve painful affects, initiate sexual intimacy, or promote greater group identification. For potential adolescent drug and alcohol abusers, efforts to improve their self-esteem and interpersonal skills enhance their capacity to refuse peer pressure.

A major role for psychiatrists is to keep parents, educators, and pediatricians better informed regarding the signs of adolescent drug use. A decline in school performance, irritability, apathy, weight loss, secrecy, or oversensitivity in response to questions about drinking or sudden changes in friends may indicate a child at risk for drug abuse. Heavy drinking in adolescence is frequently accompanied by other behavioral problems including antisocial behavior and other substance abuse. Psychiatrists can help identify high-risk groups, including children of alcoholics or children with affective illness, hyperactivity, or handicaps in an effort to help school officials target primary prevention programs.

A routine medical exam before the start of camp or school should include substance abuse screening. Use of new and sensitive tests for accurate detection of chemicals in the urine represent an advance and constitute a major aid in early detection. Marijuana use can be detected two to four weeks after use through gas chromotography and mass spectrometry. The use of these tests by pediatricians, child psychiatrists, and school health personnel may help confirm a diagnosis whenever there is question. These tests may be as useful as blood sugar levels to diagnose juvenile diabetes.

Self-help groups such as Alateen, Alatot, and activist groups such as Mothers Against Drunk Driving (MADD), provide support, dissemination of educational materials, and lobbying clout. Independently organized groups can exert strong influence. For example, a group of parents in Atlanta collectively intervened with their marijuana-abusing teenagers by providing strong external control through their exposure of local drug pushers (14). If such self-help interventions are to be successful, they must be initiated when the target group of youngsters is in grade school or junior high.

Studies on the success and cost effectiveness of school substance abuse counselors are needed. In New York, Westchester County has developed a student assistance model program in the schools that works similarly to employee assistance programs. The four components of this program include education groups for children of alcoholics, treatment or referral for abusing students, early screening of students with behavioral changes consistent with substance abuse, and cooperation with parents and community groups (15). In the 1983-84 school year, 56 percent of students were self-referred and 73 percent of all students seen were children of alcoholics or drug abusers.

Some prevention programs have been targeted toward college-age students. Small numbers of alcohol and drug abuse education programs are available on college campuses. Direct campus mailing has been described as an inexpensive technique that may enhance information dissemination to this population (16).

MASS MEDIA

Radio and television campaigns have used popular teenage figures to relate messages about prevention. For example, Brooke Shields and Michael Jackson are role models who have been active in antismoking and substance abuse campaigns. Training peer leaders for school-based lecture discussion groups is a promising extension of this approach. Mass media campaigns have increased the general public's awareness of prevention issues, but their effect on level of behavioral change is not clear. One study showed that strong appeals to fear often evoked ambivalence among targeted groups and reinforced a moral rather than medical model (17). Controversy has surrounded broadcasts of visually explicit commercials, such as the recent anti-cigarette-smoking commercial that depicts a fetus smoking, whereas others featuring prominent entertainers, such as Brooke Shields, have been well received. Research could be devised to determine the best approach for these messages. For example, it would be valuable to compare the results of anti-drug-abuse messages delivered by parental figures such as Nancy Reagan contrasted with an age peer, such as Michael Jackson, or a famous recovering person, such as Mary Tyler Moore.

New York requires bars to post warnings about drinking during pregnancy in an effort to reduce the incidence of fetal alcohol syndrome. Such efforts attempt to reach high-risk individuals where they work and play and do not involve large expense, but they are not devoid of controversy. Advertisers use mass media to increase sales of addictive substances, and substance abuse is frequently glamorized on television and in films. Some studies have shown the frequency of types of messages received through mass media and their impact on attitudes and behaviors concerning alcohol and drug abuse, but more are needed. Cafiso et al. concluded that the negative consequences of alcohol are not shown and that alcohol is generally depicted in nonproblematic ways on television (18). Commercials generally treat alcohol positively. Positive images including comraderie, relaxation, and humor are conveyed by beer commercials (19). Alcoholics may be particularly influenced by the subliminal messages in these commercials, but the negative impact this has on prevention efforts is unclear. For example, Kohn and Smart's (20) did not find that beer commercials had a strong influence on young men's beer consumption but did find a positive correlation between liquor consumption and advertisement (20).

PREVENTION AT THE WORK PLACE

Intoxication and chronic drug abuse are associated with a severe loss of employee productivity. For example, injury and illness associated with the work place, absenteeism, poor work quality, and bad morale contribute to decreased worker output. In 1980, among military personnel, 22 percent suffered work impairment secondary to alcohol use, with 77 percent of these individuals described as alcohol dependent (21). A one-third decrease in drug abuse in the military was attributed to an aggressive early detection, educational, and treatment program. The program's use of urine screens allowed for treatment after the first detection. If drugs were detected a second time, tough administrative action was taken. The core message was that drug use is no longer acceptable behavior in the military. In the business world, thousands of employee assistance programs have been developed as companies have realized the potential cost effectiveness of primary prevention.

The disease model of alcoholism promotes better acceptance of the problem employee. Holistic concepts including general health promotion, stress reduction, and enhancement of job satisfaction are receiving serious attention. Interventions have ranged from broad-based primary prevention efforts to early detection, referral, and treatment systems. Preemployment drug screens are now being used routinely in the National Football League and major league baseball teams. The increased sensitivity and accuracy of drug screen technology has increased its usefulness, especially among captive audiences such as the military and teenagers applying for a driver's license.

The use of these tests raises ethical issues such as an individual's right to privacy versus prevention and treatment for the good of the larger group. A recent Supreme Court decision upheld the right of schools to act in loco parentis and allowed searches of students suspected of possessing drugs. Professional sports teams and the Olympics now require athletes to give urine samples before events. It may well be that society will increasingly demand use of drug screens, especially in jobs in which the hazards produced by impairment are high, such as among airline pilots, surgeons, and school bus drivers. The role of urine testing and early detection of drug problems in schools may evolve from a voluntary measure into a policy of requirement. While the need for screening is higher in schools with high drug use, periodic drug screening may be a cost-effective intervention at primary, secondary, and tertiary levels of prevention. In the workplace, management's ability to skillfully detect and confront impaired employees is also essential to early intervention. When union and management work together with an employee assistance professional, confrontation techniques are especially effective. Confrontational strategy works by providing a constructive crisis for the problem employee. Employees are offered treatment and rehabilitation while progressive actions are outlined that would increase the personal cost of abusing substances. Early confrontation is often all that is necessary, but if necessary, additional disciplinary measures may deepen the crisis (22, 23).

SOCIAL POLICY AND LEGAL EFFORTS

Social policy and legal efforts on many fronts attempt to limit the availability of alcohol and illegal substances. The greater the availability of any addictive substance, the greater the craving for it and the higher the use. Alcohol is presently the most readily available, cheapest, legal, and widely used substance of abuse. Efforts to limit the influx of illegal substances is a constant struggle because such huge profits can be made from the sale of drugs. Illegal drug use is tied to market values of cost, availability, and quality. Drug profits may be a significant proportion of local economies, both in this country and abroad, and powerful organized crime czars continue to control drug traffic. Strategies to control the drug problem, including the destruction of crops (for example, spraying of marijuana fields with paraquat in Mexico), require intergovernmental cooperation.

Limiting the availability of alcohol may be approached on many fronts. Price manipulation, outward availability, hours of sale, and age restriction policies have been hotly debated in the literature. Methodical difficulties in the research of this area remain. Increasing the price of alcohol and cigarettes by taxation has been recommended. In New York, Governor Mario Cuomo has proposed increased taxes on alcohol to be used for treatment of alcoholics. This reflects a belief that heavy consumers should bear more of the financial burden of prevention and treatment in society.

Countries such as Sweden use price increases as a means to control alcohol consumption, although a consumption-price correlation has not been convincingly demonstrated (24). Evaluation of a taxation policy as a means to control consumption should include all alcoholic beverages. For example, increasing only the tax on distilled spirits may increase beer sales.

Discussion of the rate of alcohol consumption in relationship to the availability of commercial beverage outlets in a community also provokes controversy. Smart suggested that greater income and urbanism is a better measure of consumption than general availability (25). Particular subgroups may tend to use certain types of outlets (26). Forbidding grocery stores to sell alcohol and the banning of hotel room refrigerator dispensers are examples of efforts to reduce exposure of recovering alcoholics and teenagers to marketing pressures that increase the availability.

The importance of limiting alcohol consumption is underscored by the positive correlation between per capita alcohol consumption and rate of liver cirrhosis. Colon et al. (27) predicted the liver cirrhosis mortality in 50 states and the District of Columbia by alcohol consumption rates. The correlation of alcohol consumption rates with social problems seems intuitive, but has been confirmed by research (28). The pendulum is swinging back toward raising the legal drinking age. Evidence has been cited from studies in Michigan and Illinois showing that raising that minimal drinking age has decreased teenage motor vehicle accidents and deaths (29). Problems sometimes arise when adjacent states have different minimal age requirements. Several states are now looking at proposals to raise drinking age in order to avoid loosing federal highway funds. Other traffic safety laws and policies such as required seat belts, air bags, bike helmets, and crash-proof cars can prevent alcohol-related morbidity and mortality.

HIGH-RISK GROUPS

Goodwin et al. (30) found strong evidence of a genetic factor in the etiology of some forms of alcoholism. Individuals adopted out soo after birth who had one biological parent with alcoholism had higher rates of drinking problems than and three times the divorce rates of control adoptees. In families with a biological parent with alcoholism and one brother adopted out while the other stayed at home, both brothers had similar incidence of alcoholism, approximately four times greater than the general population. This demonstrates that taking the biologically vulnerable child out of the alcoholic household does not reduce risk (31).

Distinguishing familial versus nonfamilial alcoholism has important prognostic and prevention ramifications. Awareness of high family risk for heart disease led to efforts to reduce risk factors such as cigarette smoking, obesity, hypertension, and cholesterol in this high-risk group of children. Similarly, identification of individuals at high risk for developing alcoholism could lead to education about alternative alcohol-free life-styles and be helpful in prevention. Attempts are being made to characterize familial versus nonfamilial alcoholics. Our group found that familial alcoholics have an earlier onset of problem drinking, more severe social consequences, less consistently stable family involvement, poorer academic and social performance in school, more antisocial behavior, and a poorer outcome in treatment (32).

Children of alcoholics have been called "the hidden tragedy" and "the neglected problem" (33, 34). They are exposed to both genetic and environmental factors that put them at higher risk. Understanding protective factors may be helpful, and intervention with these children at an early age may be beneficial.

One approach is to learn more about the connection between family disorganization, alcoholism, and emotional disturbance in children. Children of alcoholics often deal with emotional stigma, alienation, estrangement and isolation from others they see living a more normal family life. Alcoholic parents are frequently inconsistent and emotionally depriving. The nonalcoholic parent's role takes on an added importance for the child. These children may assume inappropriate nurturing and protective roles within the family. Sexual identity roles are often confused, and divisive splits in the family develop secondary to feelings of anger and abandonment.

Understanding the experience of being a child of an alcoholic helps to better understand the challenge of helping prevent or treat the problem. Growing up in an inconsistent household in which the parents may sometimes be kind and loving and other times punitive and withdrawn leads to a distrust of authority figures and a greater tendency to depend on peers or no one. Siblings have to care for each other as well as take care of their parents, and they tend to pick friends from similarly troubled families. They are afraid to bring home friends who don't have families with problems similar to their own. This peer group grows up protesting their parent's behavior, trying to be different, but ending up with the same problems. It is not surprising then that they do not trust doctors, teachers, nurses, or other professionals who represent authority figures. It also explains why self-help groups, group therapy, and family approaches are especially helpful. This explains why Alcoholics Anonymous, Alateen, Alanon, Drugs Anonymous, school-based support groups, and groups for adult children of alcoholics have wide appeal and effectiveness .Alcohol treatment programs are beginning to design special three-generational counseling programs for the children of alcoholic patients and their children.

Attempts are being made to characterize the natural history of various forms of alcoholism. The natural history of alcohol and drug abuse may show a substantial degree of instability over time. Alder reported on sequential stepping-stone use of alcohol, cigarettes, marijuana, and harder drugs (35). Prospective longitudinal studies of high-risk groups, along with cohorts of different ages, may help to identify the psychosocial factors that promote or deter drinking and substance abuse. McCord et al.found aggressive and impulsive problems in adolescents who had future drinking problems (28). Beardslee and Vaillant reported prospective longitudinal data, however, that suggest there may be no personality style predictive of alcoholism (36).

With the development of multiaxial diagnosis in the *DSM-III*, research has increased on the correlation of other psychopathology with alcohol and substance abuse. Correlation with rates of depression, psychosis, anxiety, and hyperactivity with addictive behaviors has involved extensive epidemiological studies. In 1974 Winokur suggested a depression-spectrum disease, characterized by an early onset of depression predominately in female relatives, with an increased frequency in alcohol and antisocial behavior in male relatives (36). This suggests the possibility of genetic vulnerability to mental illness that may take the form of alcohol and substance abuse. Cloninger et al. cited evidence that alcoholism, sociopathy, and depression are genetically distinct (38). Cadoret et al. also recently suggested a specificity of inheritance of antisocial and alcoholic conditions (39).

Loranger and Tulis (40) reported that borderline patients have a two to three times increase in their family history of alcoholism compared with bipolar or schizophrenic patients. Bohman et al. reported on various somatization disorders and their correlations with primary versus secondary alcoholism in fathers (41). An association between hyperactive syndrome and children of alcoholics has been suggested (42). A retrospective study of primary versus secondary alcoholics reported higher evidence of a childhood minimal brain disorder in primary alcoholics (43). Tarter, in a study of primary alcoholics, reported a higher percentage of minimal brain damage and poorer performance on neuropsychological tests in that population (44). One-third to one-half of psychiatric hospital admissions have been reported to have complicating drug abuse problems (45). So-called dual diagnosis patients with major psychiatric illness and alcohol and substance abuse are becoming more common in inpatient psychiatric drug abuse centers. Prevention and early treatment of other disorders may help prevent substance dependency.

SPECIAL POPULATIONS

Studies by psychiatrists, sociologists, and anthropologists have delineated cross-cultural issues in alcoholism. Women, the elderly, Hispanics, Native Americans, Blacks, homosexuals, multihandicapped individuals, and the developmentally disabled are subgroups that function in a social, cultural, and political matrix that must be taken into account when designing primary prevention programs.

Women

Awareness of alcohol and substance abuse among women is increasing. Social and psychological etiological factors are more often associated with women who have marital problems; are divorced or separated; or suffer from role confusion, low self-esteem, or sexual and obstetrical difficulties. The link between feelings of alienation and alcohol use is greater among women, although single employed women with higher education, curiously may have higher rates of alcohol consumption than those of other groups of women (46, 47).

Stress that is related to conflicting expectations of women in society may also play a part. In one Baltimore study, being married or widowed, having lower educational attainment, and having less egalitarian sexual attitudes was associated with lower alcohol consumption (48). Being married to an alcoholic spouse may increase risks for alcohol problems. Women are more often prescribed psychoactive substances by physicians who may unwittingly foster pharmacological solutions to stress. Prevention and treatment strategies have been looking to facilitate better stress management and increased assertive and coping skills among women. The association between heavy alcohol usage during pregnancy and birth defects is fairly well established. The effects of the use of any amount of alcohol whatsoever during pregnancy is still unclear. However, at this time alcohol abstinence is recommended.

Elderly

Awareness of alcohol abuse among the elderly is also growing. Social, cultural and psychological factors interplay to make detection and prevention of the problem difficult. Institutionalized bias and prejudice may obscure the diagnosis among the elderly. Criteria for the diagnosis of alcoholism in the elderly may have to be modified. Repeated unexplained falls, confusion, and self-neglect may be a tip-off to a hidden alcohol abuse problem (49). Alcohol abuse generally decreases with advancing age; however, a subset of individuals may become problem drinkers after a life-long abstinence (50). Losses such as retirement or loss of a spouse, social isolation, and financial limitations play a role. Alcohol abuse among the elderly takes a greater toll on their cognitive and medical health. Alcoholism is seen in 15 percent or more of older individuals presenting to psychiatrists with pathology ranging from depression to acute psychiatric states (51). Usual motivations for treatment, such as threat of job loss, premature death, and family confrontation, are often limited (52).

Hispanics and Native Americans

Rates of alcoholism among Hispanics and Native Americans appear to be high (53). A tailored approach is required if ethnic groups are to have access to treatment. Familiarity, proximity, communication and acceptance enhances availability to treatment and the success of prevention strategies. An understanding of culturally accepted modes of treatment would be helpful in characterizing natural coping channels. Alcoholics Anonymous concepts may not be acceptable across all cultures. For example, the Navajo Indian may find them too personal and Costa Ricans find their concept of surrender to be socially unacceptable (54). Ideas about manhood and group status are often integrated with alcoholic beverages. Different cultures hold different views about the effects of alcohol and drugs on interpersonal relationships and smooth social or economic functioning. Mexican Americans experience a strong sense of family identification that may heighten the experience of shame for an alcoholic. In some cultures, intrusion into the family system may promote marked resistance from the patient and family (53).

Blacks

The drinking problems of Blacks may become evident earlier in life due to the prevailing economic and social bias and possible genetic factors. Blacks may suffer more severe medical problems, such as cirrhosis in younger age groups, and more severe legal problems due to binge-pattern drinking (55). The role of alcohol and substance abuse associated with the high rate of Black homicide needs to be clarified (56).

Homosexuals

Homosexuality, though not causally related, has been associated with high risk of alcohol and substance abuse. Social life at bars, social stigma and bias, and the use of alcohol as a social disinhibitor are factors involved with abuse (57). Increased awareness and a mobilization of the gay community to promote alternative lifestyles, as has been seen in the recent Acquired Immunity Deficiency syndrome (AIDS) epidemic, also may be beneficial with substance abuse problems. Treatment of addictions may also reduce the spread of AIDS, through both self-restraint and reduction in the use of dirty needles.

Multihandicapped

Rehabilitation centers that work with multihandicapped patients report that 25 to 30 percent of their clients abuse alcohol alone or in combination with other drugs. For several reasons, the disabled are at a high risk of becoming substance abusers. They often have easy access to alcohol and drugs because staff and families will facilitate their use or at least not object, out of guilt or a sense of futility. Disabled people often feel frustrated and angry at being dependent, socially isolated, and discriminated against by the rest of society. As a group, they are vulnerable to feelings of depression, anxiety, self-hatred, low motivation, and low self-esteem, and they often undertake self-medication with alcohol and other substances.

The blind and deaf have special problems that include denial of the existence of alcohol and substance problems within their community, the fear of being stigmatized, and the lack of adequate signs in sign language to symbolize drunkeness or sobriety. Treatment facilities generally do not have counselors or professionals trained in sign language. Patients with spinal cord disability and alcoholism are common, probably as a result of the accidents caused by alcohol. Spinal cord injury patients may have physical problems that are aggravated by substance abuse, including decubitus ulcers caused by immobility, poor nutrition, and sexual dysfunction. Many sustained their injuries while intoxicated and continue to use alcohol to cope with their situation. The Veterans

Administration Hospital at Long Beach, California, has a program geared to treat the spinal-cord-injured alcoholic that combines physical rehabilitation, group psychotherapy, and recovery groups such as Alcoholics Anonymous and Narcotics Anonymous.

Developmentally Disabled

The developmentally disabled, alcoholic, mentally retarded patients with an IQ of 60 to 85 are concrete, are easily manipulated, and have difficulty learning from experience. They may find the neighborhood bar to be a warm, nonjudgmental place where they feel accepted and part of a group. Since deinstitutionalization, many mentally retarded people living in the community lack necessary skills for positive socialization. They turn to alcohol and substance abuse as an easy solution. It is hard for them to learn about alcohol in programs designed for those with a higher IQ. Therefore, they need special support and help to overcome alcohol dependency.

BIOLOGICAL AND BASIC RESEARCH

Recently attention has been focused on the search for biological markers of illness in schizophrenia, depression, anxiety, and alcohol and substance abuse. In the long run, basic research may provide the key to prevention of certain forms of alcohol and substance abuse. Early identification of high-risk individuals may provide the most effective primary prevention intervention. Controversy surrounds the idea that individuals are attempting to self-medicate themselves when abusing substances. For some addicted people there may be a special fit between the brain and the drug, and they try different drugs until the required result is obtained. Schuckit proposed that the alcohol and substance themselves are responsible for creating prevailing moods (58). The use of certain drugs may lead to use of other more addictive substances, but this is not invariably so. Goodwin proposed a model of alcoholism in which deficient neurotransmitter activity of serotonin may be improved by alcohol intake (1). On the other hand, excess production of morphine-like alkaloids in the brain by exposure to alcohol may facilitate alcohol addiction (59). In stimulant abuse, undocumented histories of minimal brain damage should be sought. These approaches may provide means of better pharmacological manipulation of tolerance and dependence in high-risk individuals.

Recent studies have shown a great individual variation in the response to ethanol in animals and in humans. This includes their central nervous system sensitivity, development of tolerance and dependence, metabolic rate, drinking behavior, and susceptibility to alcoholic cirrhosis and organicity (60). An important experimental tool has been the development of strains of animals selectively bred with alcohol preference. These pure strains of animals may provide better models for understanding the neurobiological and biochemical correlates of normal and abnormal alcohol drinking behavior (60). Human metabolism of alcohol may vary thricefold across individuals even after correction for body weight, diet, and other environmental factors. Research on the properties of the metabolising isoenzyme alcohol dehydrogenase has shown different kinetic properties across individuals and racial groups. A genetic absence of a variant of this enzyme may explain the alcohol flush reaction, which includes facial flushing, tachycardia, nausea, vomiting, and hypertension resulting from alcohol abuse that occurs in 50 percent of Japanese individuals. The flush response may be protective against alcoholism in Oriental cultures (61). Metabolism rates may help to identify individuals susceptible to abnormal tolerance and dependency.

Used acutely, alcohol makes cell wall membranes more plastic and fluid. Chronic alcohol intake renders cell walls more rigid. There may be a genetic organ sensitivity to chronic alcohol intake. The hippocampus and the locus ceruleus are brain areas extremely sensitive to alcohol (60).

Further understanding of basic science issues involving interactions of alcohol and nutrition, hormones, neurotransmitters, and platelet enzymes is needed. Identification of sensitive enzyme tests such as the blood gamma-glutamyltranspeptidase, which is elevated in more than 50 percent of alcoholics, and characteristic blood profiles may provide early indicators of problem drinking in individuals who are still socially and medically without definite stigmata (62). Platelet markers such as monoamine oxidase inhibition and serotonin reuptake have been studied (63).

A recent Danish study indicated that sons of alcoholics generate greater increases in slow wave alpha activity on electroencephalograms after drinking alcohol than do sons of nonalcoholics (64). Begleiter described a characteristic P300 wave attenuation on the evoked potential found in alcoholics and sons of alcoholics that may provide a trait marker for alcoholism. The P300 wave is thought to be a characteristic of the decreased reaction to novel experience and is related to a hippocampal deficit. Prospective studies are needed to determine whether evoked potential could discriminate those at highest risk (65). Schuckit reported a decreased subjective response to alcohol in sons of alcoholics compared with controls (66). Attempts to use more sophisticated multiaxial electographic beam studies may provide characteristic patterns of high risk.

Better understanding of these basic neurophysiological and biochemical mechanisms may help us to identify what is genetically transmitted and how this may interact with the neuropsychological characteristics of the disease.

CONCLUSION

Diverse approaches exist for the prevention of alcohol and substance abuse, and research is needed in many areas. While primary prevention efforts have been undertaken by health educators, by law enforcement officials, and through laws and policies developed by governmental bodies, a cohesive program has yet to be developed. Exciting research on genetic markers in high-risk individuals; the special needs of a variety of ethnic groups; and the opportunity for psychiatrists to work with patients, their families, community groups, and policy makers are all areas that depend on expanded funding for research. Policy makers and the general public, with help from psychiatric experts on primary prevention in alcohol and substance abuse, have challenging decisions to make regarding funding for research on a problem that has plagued humanity for centuries.

REFERENCES

1. Goodwin WD: Alcoholism and genetics. Arch Gen Psychiatry 42:171-174, 1985
2. Robins LN, Helzer JE, Weissman MM, et al: Lifetime prevalence of specific psychiatric disorders in three sites. Arch Gen Psychiatry 41:949-958, 1984
3. Myers JK, Weissman MM, Tischler GL, et al: Six-month prevalence of psychiatric disorder in three communities. Arch Gen Psychiatry 41:958-967, 1984
4. University of Michigan Institute for Social Research Newsletter, winter 1984
5. Substance Use Among New York State Public and Private School Students in Grades 7 Through 12, 1983. New York State Division of Substance Abuse Services, September 1984
6. Gold MS: 1-800--COCAINE. New York, Bantam Books, 1984
7. Korcok M: Strategies explored for treating cocaine abuse. AMA News 28 (44):15-16, 1985
8. Zucker R, Harford T: Natural study of the demography of adolescent drinking practices in 1980. J Stud Alcohol 44

(6):974-985, 1983
9. West LJ, Maxwell DS, Noble EP, et al: Alcoholism. Ann Intern Med 100:405-416, 1984
10. Niven GR: Alcoholism--A problem in perspective. JAMA 252:1912-1914, 1984.
11. Fifth Special Report to the U.S. Congress on Alcohol and Health From the Secretary of Health and Human Services (Publication No. ADM 84-1291). U.S. Department of Health and Human Services, 1984
12. Goodstadt M. Sheppard M: Three approaches to alcohol education. J Stud Alcohol 44:362-380, 1983.
13. Johnson CA, Graham JW, Hansen WB: Drug Use by Peer Leaders. Presented at the annual meeting of the American Psychological Association, Los Angeles, 1981
14. Griffen JB: Some psychodynamic considerations in the treatment of drug abuse in early adolescence. J Am Acad Child Psychiatry 20:159-166, 1981
15. Chambers J, Morehouse E: A cooperative model for preventing alcohol and drug abuse. NASSP Bulletin, January 1983
16. McCarty S, Poore M, Mill K, et al: Direct mail techniques and the prevention of alcohol related problems among college students. J Stud Alcohol 44: 162-190, 1983
17. Mider PA: Failures in alcoholism in drug dependenc prevention and learning from the past. Am Psychol 39:183-184, 1984
18. Cafiso J, Goodstadt MS, Garlington WK, et al: Television portrayal of alcohol and other beverages. J Stud Alcohol 43:1232-1243, 1982
19. Finn AT, Strickland DE: A content analysis of beverage alcohol advertising. II. Television advertising. J Stud Alcohol 43:964-989, 1982
20. Kohn PM, Smart RG: The impact of television advertising on alcohol consumption: an experiment. J Stud Alcohol 45:295-301, 1984
21. Bart MR: Prevalence and consequences of alcohol use among U.S. military personnel, 1980. J Stud Alcohol 43:1097-1107, 1982
22. Trice H, Beyer J, Hunt R: Evaluating implementation of a job-based alcoholism policy. J Stud Alcohol 39: 448-465, 1978
23. Trice HM, Beyer JM: Work-related outcomes of the constructive, confrontation strategy in a job-based alcoholism program. J Stud Alcohol 45:393-404, 1984
24. Levy D, Sheflin N: New evidence on controlling alcohol use through price. J Stud Alcohol 44:929-937, 1983
25. Smart R: The relationship of availability of alcoholic beverages

to per capita consumption and alcoholism rates. J Stud Alcohol 38:891-896, 1977

26. Rabow J, Watt SR: Alcohol availability, alcohol beverage sales and alcohol-related problems. J Stud Alcohol 43:767-801, 1982
27. Colon I, Cutter HSG, Jones WC: Prediction of alcoholism from alcohol availability, alcohol consumption and demographic data. J Stud Alcohol 43:1199-1213 1982
28. McCord W, McCord J, Gudeman J: Origin of Alcoholism. Stanford, CA, Stanford University Press, 1960
29. Wagernaar AC, Douglass RL: An evaluation of the changes in the legal drinking age in Michigan, summary of principle findings: the raised drinking age in Michigan. Bottom Line, Lansing 4:16-17, 1980
30. Goodwin D, Schulsinger F, Moller N, et al: Drinking problems in adopted and nonadopted sons of alcoholics. Arch Gen Psychiatry 31:164-169, 1984
31. Goodwin DW, Schulsinger F, Hermansen L, et al: Alcohol problems in adoptees raised apart from alcoholic biological parents. Arch Gen Psychiatry 28:238-243, 1973
32. Frances RJ, Tim S, Bucky S: Studies of familial and non-familial alcoholism. Arch Gen Psychiatry 37:564-566, 1980
33. el-Guebaly N, Offord D: The offspring of alcoholics: a critical review. Am J Psychiatry 134:357-365, 1977
34. Slobada S: The children of alcoholics: a neglected problem. Hosp Community Psychiatry 25:605-606, 1974
35. Alder I, Kandell DB: Cross cultural perspectives on developmental stages in adolescent drug use. J Stud Alcohol 42:701-715, 1981
36. Beardslee NR, Vaillant AE: Prospective prediction of alcoholics and psychopathology. J Stud Alcohol 45:500-503, 1984
37. Winokur GA, Cadoret R, Dorzab JA, et al: The division of depressive illness into depression spectrum disease and pure depressive illness. International Pharmacopsychiatry 9:5-13, 1974
38. Cloninger RC, Reich T, Wetzel R: Alcoholism and affective disorders: familial associations and genetic models, in Alcoholism and Affective Disorders. Edited by Goodwin CK, Erickson CK. Jamaica, NY: Spectrum Publications, 1979
39. Cadoret RJ, O'Gorman TW, Throughton E, et al: Alcoholism and antisocial personality. Arch of Gen Psychiatry 42:161-167, 1985
40. Loranger AN, Tulis EH: Family history of alcoholism in borderline personality disorder. Arch Gen Psychiatry 42:153-157, 1985
41. Bohman M, Cloninger R, Knorring AL, et al: An adoption

study of somatoform disorders. III. Cross fostering analysis and genetic relationship to alcoholism and community. Arch Gen Psychiatry 41:872-878, 1984

42. Goodwin DW, Schulsinger F, Hermansen L, et al: Alcoholism and the hyperactive child syndrome. J Nerv Ment Dis 110:345-353, 1975

43. Obaldia RE, Parsons OA: Relationship of neuropsychological performance to first-degree alcoholism and self-presented symptoms of childhood MBD. J Stud Alcohol 45:386-392, 1984

44. Tarter RE, Alterman AL: Neuropsychological deficits in alcoholics: etiological considerations. J Stud Alcohol 45:1-9, 1984

45. Crowley T, Chesluk D, Hart R: Drug and alcohol abuse among psychiatric admissions. Arch Gen Psychiatry 30:13-20, 1974

46. Camar R, Fitzgerald B, Halzren C: Alienation and drinking motivation among adolescent females. J Pers Soc Psychol 44:1021-1024, 1983

47. Holch SE, Warren CW, Smith JC, et al: Alcohol consumption among Mexican Americans and Anglo women: results of a survey along the U.S.-Mexican border. J Stud Alcohol 45:149-154, 1984

48. Celentano DD, McQueen DV: Alcohol consumption patterns among women in Baltimore. J Stud Alcohol 45:355-358, 1984

49. Watts JP: Alcohol problems in the elderly. J Am Geriatr Society 29:151-154, 1981

50. Christopherson VA, Esher NC, Bainton BR: Reasons for drinking among the elderly in rural Arizona. J Stud Alcohol 45:417-423, 1984

51. Pattee J: Uncovering the elderly "hidden alcoholic." Geriatrics 37:145-146, 1982

52. Schuckit M: A clinical review of alcohol, alcoholism and the elderly patient. J Clin Psychiatry 43:396-399, 1982

53. Paine H: Attitudes and patterns of alcohol use among Mexican Americans: implications for services delivery. J Stud Alcohol 38:544-553, 1977

54. Favazza A: Alcohol and special populations. J Stud Alcohol 9:1981-1998, 1981

55. Benjamin R, Benjamin M: Sociocultural correlates of Black drinking. J Stud Alcohol 9:241-245, 1981

56. The Role of the Core Mental Health Professions in Preventing and Reducing the Incidence of Black Homicide. Rockville, MD, National Institute of Mental Health Center for Studies of Minority Group Mental Health

57. Small E, Leach B: Counseling homosexual alcoholics. J Stud Alcohol 30:2077-2085, 1977

58. Schuckit MA: Alcoholism and other psychiatric disorders. Hosp Community Psychiatry 34:1022-1026, 1983
59. Jeffoate WJ, Herbert M, Cullen MH, et al: Prevention of effects of alcohol intoxication by Naloxone. Lancet 2:1157-1158, 1979
60. Report of the 1983 Research Planning Panel. Rockville, MD, National Institute of Alcohol Abuse and Alcoholism
61. Schwittes SY, Johnson RC, McClean GE, et al: Alcohol use and the flushing response in different rural and ethnic groups. J Stud Alcohol 43:1254-1262, 1982
62. Trill E, Kristenson H, Fex G: Alcohol-related problems in middle age men with elevated serum gamma glutamyltransferase: a preventive medical investigation. J Stud Alcohol 45:302-309, 1984
63. Kent TA, Campbell JR, Goodwin DW: Blood platelet uptake of serotonin in chronic alcoholics. Lancet, in press
64. Pollack VE, Volavka J, Goodwin DW, et al: The EEG after alcohol in men at risk for alcoholism. Arch Gen Psychiatry 40:857-861, 1983
65. Begleiter H, Porjesz B, Chou CL, et al: P300 and stimulus incentive value. Psychophysiology, 1:95-101, 1983
66. Schuckit MA: Subjective responses to alcohol of sons of alcoholic and control subjects. Arch Gen Psychiatry 41:879-884, 1984

7

Primary Prevention of Homicide

Kenneth Tardiff, M.D., M.P.H.

7

Primary Prevention of Homicide

Approximately 23,000 people are murdered each year in the United States. Homicide accounts for more than one percent of total deaths each year, with some segments of the population being at greater risk than others. Risk of death by homicide is increased among the young, male, Black and Hispanic members of our society (1-14). This deprivation of life and its impact on family and friends of victims is a major public health problem deserving attention from physicians and the public. This chapter presents an outline of what we know and do not know about determinants of violence, particularly violence leading to homicide. In addition areas at which primary prevention intervention should be targeted are discussed.

DETERMINANTS OF VIOLENCE

Biological or psychological markers useful for primary prevention of violence currently do not exist, and if they did, we might not know how to use them given the complex legal, ethical, and clinical questions that would arise. The absence of a clearly identifiable biological marker for violence does not imply that research has been neglected in this area.

Brain Wave Abnormalities

Building on earlier studies in which a greater proportion of certain electroencephalogram (EEG) patterns were found among violent prisoners (15-17), Mark and Ervin (18) argued that aggressive behavior could be localized in the temporal lobe and, more specifically, in the amygdala. Since then it has beem agreed that the role of the amygdala has been overstated in the prevalence of violent behavior, and the suggestion that neurosurgical procedures be used in temporal lobe epilepsy has provoked concern in society about the use of these procedures. In a recent review, Hermann and Whitman (19) concluded that "despite the many anecdotal reports in the literature and media of alleged outbursts of violence by people with epilepsy (and temporal lobe epilepsy in particular), controlled investigations have consistently reported no overall temporal lobe epilepsy/non-temporal lobe epilepsy differences. Furthermore, the only two controlled studies among prisoners have also failed to detect elevated levels of violence or increased seriousness of crime among prisoners with epilepsy compared with prisoners without epilepsy" (p. 474).

Where differences have been found, they have often been related to confounding variables such as socioeconomic status, sex, age, and early environment. This does not exclude gross brain dysfunction as a contributor to violence but merely points out that no specific deficit has been demonstrated. For example, Lewis (20) found that extremely violent boys in a correctional school had an increased occurrence of neurological and psychiatric problems including grossly abnormal EEGs.

Genetics

In the area of genetic inheritance, recent twin studies found increased criminal behavior in monozygotic twins compared with dizygotic twins (21). However, given that twins in these studies often shared the same environmental as well as genetic backgrounds, investigators turned to studies of separately adopted twins. In two such studies in Scandinavia (22, 23) no support was found for a genetic basis for homicidal behavior, but some support was found for a genetic association for crimes involving property. In terms of specific genetic defects or markers, there has been great interest in research over the past two decades on sex chromosome abnormalities, particularly the XYY complement. In a number of surveys of men in prisons and other correctional institutions, XYY men were discovered to be disproportionately represented in these institutions. More recent findings (24) showing no evidence to support a relationship between violence and the XYY complement in the population at large should end this speculation.

Hormones

The role of male and female hormones in violence has been studied. For example, a number of studies (25-28) have explore the role of androgens in aggression has been explored, a significant relationship between testosterone levels and aggressive behavior has not been found. These studies have been conducted predominantly on prison populations. In women, the premenstrual syndrome (PMS) has been linked to violent crime (29). Critics, however, argue (30) that placebos and controls have not been used and other aspects of PMS interventions, such as alcohol avoidance and maintenance of a stable diet as well as individual personality characteristics have not been properly or adequately accounted for in these studies of the relationship between PMS and violence.

Neurotransmitters

Recently attention has turned to the possible role of neurotransmitters in violence. Brown et al. (31, 32) conducted two studies of men with a history of aggressive behavior. Men with a history of primary affective disorders, schizophrenia, or severe brain syndromes and those who had ingested drugs or alcohol 10 days preceding the study were excluded. Brown et al. found that a history of aggressive behavior and a history of suicidal behavior were both related to decreased cerebrospinal fluid levels of 5-hydroxyindoleacetic acid (5-HIAA). They hypothesize that altered serotonin metabolism may be a highly significant contributing factor to aggressive and suicidal behaviors in whatever diagnostic group they occur. Lidberg et al.(33) studied the cerebrospinal fluid 5-HIAA levels in men convicted of criminal homicide and men who attempted suicide and found that both of these groups had lower levels of 5-HIAA in spinal fluid than did male controls. Lidberg et al.did not, as Brown did, exclude alcoholics or patients with schizophrenia or affective illness, which may confound their results. Linnoila et al. (34) also studied violent offenders, excluding schizophrenics or those with major affective disorders but not alcoholics. All of the subjects had killed or attempted to kill with unusual cruelty. They found that impulsive offenders had significantly lower cerebrospinal fluid 5-HIAA concentrations than did nonimpulsive offenders. The nonimpulsive offenders were defined as those who had premeditated their crime. Linnolia et al. concluded that low cerebrospinal fluid 5-HIAA concentration may be a marker of impulsivity rather than of a specific type of violence, such as suicide or externally directed violence. The study of neurotransmitters holds some promise in identifying underlying mechanisms of violence, but only preliminary work has been done.

Psychiatric Diagnosis

Other researchers and I (35-41) have studied systematically the frequency of violent behavior by psychiatric patients and have determined that certain types of patients are at a higher risk of committing violence. These include the young, males, and certain diagnostic groups, depending on the type of setting studied. These studies have been useful in developing treatment policy, including the setting of staffing levels in relation to the risk of violent behavior, the need for staff education and techniques of management of violent patients, and the establishment of various levels of care both in and outside of hospital. Studies (42, 43) comparing controls with murderers and nonviolent offenders on dimensions such as psychiatric diagnosis or batteries of psychological tests have not been useful in the prediction of the long term risk of violent behavior or the prevention of homicide.

Clinically, we can assess the short-term probability of serious violent behavior when deciding whether to admit a patient to hospital. Problems arise when we try to predict whether a patient will kill someone upon discharge from the hospital. A frequent scenario involves a paranoid schizophrenic who is assaultive or seriously homicidal, is admitted to the hospital, responds to neuroleptic medication, manifests less psychopathology in terms of delusional thinking (or at least does not talk about it), and appears ready for placement in the community. Staff are rightly concerned about noncompliance with medication once he leaves the hospital, which would result in increased delusional thinking and possibly homicide. A solution to this problem is found in state laws providing for mandatory outpatient treatment. This may be preferable to lifelong psychiatric hospitalization. Unfortunately, there are problems with implementing these laws, because mental health professionals do not view themselves as police pursuing patients who refuse treatment. Mental health professionals also have realistic concerns about entering the residence of a patient who may be homicidal and armed.

Another major problem for mental health professionals lies in Tarasoff-like court decisions (44), which place a responsibility on therapists to protect intended victims of violence or homicide. Discharging this responsibility creates problems for the therapist, because even in the face of an expressed threat it is not possible to predict accurately that a person will kill another person. Additional concerns are how to warn a victim, issues of confidentiality, avoiding needless distress caused by inappropriate warnings, and recognizing that the intended victim and police may have limited abilities to prevent an intended homicide.

Child Abuse

Reducing the incidence and prevalence of child abuse may be an effective method of preventing violence and homicide. It is known that being abused as a child is often a precursor to being an abusive parent, and abused children are often involved in juvenile delinquency and other forms of violence (45-47). Certain characteristics are found regularly among parents who are at higher risk of abusing their children (47-50). These include being a single parent; being a young parent, especially a teenaged one; being at a poverty level and having little or no social support; and having a child who is handicapped or sick. There is evidence (51, 52) that abused children grow up without role models to teach them appropriate control of anger and that this occurs from a very early age, possibly before age 2. Gladston (51) recommended intervention before the age of 18 months to enhance the possibility of modifying a child's later violent behavior. Programs of primary prevention (53) involving individual and family group therapies have been aimed at parents thought to be at high risk for child abuse. In addition to psychotherapeutic preventive measures, social support and remediation of poverty are prime considerations for prevention efforts.

Alcohol and Drug Abuse

Alcohol and drugs have definite proven links with violence. A number of reviews of studies (54-57) demonstrate a persistently high proportion of alcohol use in both victims and perpetrators of violence. This is particularly evident in violence associated with interpersonal disputes involving family or friends. Alcohol's role may be to decrease inhibition. The inebriated victim becomes verbally or physically abusive and provocative. In response to this provocation, the assailant, also experiencing decreased inhibition, acts rather than restrains himself or herself. In a Manhattan study (14), alcohol was found to be more often associated with homicides involving interpersonal disputes rather than in other criminal activities such as drug dealing or robbery. Drug abuse has been found to be related to violence in a direct, pharmacologic way. Drugs involved include amphetamines (56, 58), phencyclidine (59), sedatives and minor tranquilizers (60, 61). The first two classes of drugs contribute to violence through delusional thinking, perceptional distortions, and increased psychomotor activity, whereas the latter classes of drugs decrease inhibition and increase impulsivity. Opioid drug abuse is related to violence indirectly, not through a primary psychopharmacologic effect. Narcotics play a key role because of the high incidence of criminal activities involved in obtaining these drugs. In a number of studies (14, 62, 63) narcotics have been found in the blood of homicide victims. The finding in Manhattan (14) that one-third of male homicide victims died in drug-related homicides is probably true for a number of large cities.

Firearms

Firearms play an important part in homicides, for they can turn what might have been an assault into a homicide. Nationally, Jason et al. (64) found that more than two-thirds of homicides, in the period from 1976 to 1979, involved firearms. There has been a significant increase in the number of homicides associated with firearms since the beginning of this century, and particularly since 1960 (3). Yet determining whether this increase is due to increased availability of firearms is complex and not easily ascertained. Some measures of availability of firearms have included information about the manufacture, import, and sales of guns. Yet imports are not measured accurately and there is little available data on exports or the rate at which all guns are removed from circulation. Data about the general availability of guns may not reveal much about the relationship of firearms to homicide (65-68).

Since there is doubt about defining availability and difficulty in linking availability data to homicide rates, some researchers have turned to evaluating the impact of gun control legislation on violence and homicide rates. Findings concerning state gun control legislation are not homogenous. The Gun Control Act of 1968 was found to have no effect on homicide in New York and Boston (69). However, both the Bartley-Fox Amendment and the District of Columbia's Firearms Control Act of 1975 have been shown to be related to a decrease of homicides involving firearms (70, 71). What we do not know is how available guns are to criminals in the illegitimate market and whether their use in homicide-related crimes would be decreased by gun control legislation.

The Role of Law in Primary Prevention

Regarding deliberate, intentional criminal violence, the deterrence effect of the law may be considered as a primary prevention strategy. Most studies on deterrence have analyzed variations in crime rates and sanctions between geographic areas. Capital punishment has been proposed as a preventive measure, most notably by Ehrlich (72). Using data from the Federal Bureau of Investigation Uniform Crime Reports, he supported his hypothesis that executions can have the effect of preventing homicides. However, a National Academy of Sciences study (73) reviewed his and other studies and found that the evidence did not support the deterrence theory. Furthermore it was found that crime rates may in turn influence sanctions.

As a means of secondary prevention, it has been found that the effect of simple incarceration of a prisoner results in a decrease in crime rates (74). Moore et al. (75) gave a qualified endorsement to selective arrest and prosecution of offenders with a history of previous serious and dangerous behavior. An improved information system would be needed to accomplish this. The concept is based on retribution for the serious offense rather than on prediction of future dangerous behavior. The authors admit that even if ethical and legal considerations can be addressed, a far greater challenge is the prevention of less serious offenses such as domestic assault and persistent disorderly conduct. The deterrent effects of arrest for domestic assault rather than counseling or ordering a suspect to leave has been proven effective in a research project in Minneapolis (76). Arrested subjects manifested significantly less subsequent violence than did other subjects in the study. This contradicts past views of the role of police in domestic violence. It should be noted that counseling in the form of crisis intervention may be more appropriate than arrest in cases of interpartner abuse, that is, cases not entailing unilateral violence toward a spouse. Such techniques have been outlined in a recent article by Felthous and may be considered a strategy for secondary prevention of domestic violence or primary prevention of homicide (77).

Television and Other Media

Television viewing and other mass media have been suspected as causal factors in violence.In a recent report (78) by the NIMH on entertainment programming, approximately 2,500 studies conducted since 1970 were reviewed. Most of these studies were found to demonstrate a relationship between televised violence and later aggressive behavior. Freedman (79) was critical of the NIMH report, pointing out that few of the studies reviewed concerned the relatively long-term effects of television or did not involve natural settings. In his review of field experiments and correlational studies, he concluded that there is a consistent small correlation between television violence and aggressiveness but there is little convincing evidence from natural settings that viewing television violence causes people to be more aggressive.

Not addressed is the role of news reports depicting violence, assassinations, and other murders, or the effect of motion pictures and television music videos on the general increasing level of violence in the United States. These may be reflected in specific acts which, at times, bear an uncanny resemblance to what has been portrayed on the screen. Also not addressed is the use of short television commercials or extended programs to educate and promote prosocial behavior.

Social Factors

There is evidence that social control of crime by members of society other than law enforcement officials may deter violence and other crime. Shotland and Goodstein (80) found that the number of bystanders available for surveillance and intervention may prevent the commission of crime, and, in turn, fear of crime may reduce the number of bystanders available for surveillance. This suggests that under certain circumstances crime causes crime and further implies that an important factor in the social control of crime is the relative balance between an offender's fear of surveillance and a bystander's fear of crime. The relative strength of each of these forces determines whether a neighborhood will be either safe or hostile and dangerous in terms of violence. This hypothesis is consistent with the findings of Messner and Tardiff (81), who analyzed the social ecology of homicide patterns in New York City. This study used the "routine activities" approach to explain direct-contact predatory violations. Direct-contact predatory violations have three components: an offender motivated to commit the violation; a suitable target to be victimized by the offender; and the absence of guardians capable of preventing the violation. This study found that the probability of "capable guardians" being present was related to the incidence of homicide.

Racial Versus Economic Factors

The high rates of homicide and other criminal violence affect the Black population as victims and perpetrators more than they affect the White population as such. Some authors (82) have hypothesized that Blacks live in a violent subculture, whereas others (83) have found that for domestic homicide, no difference exists in homicide rates between Blacks and Whites when socioeconomic status is controlled. There is a definite economic relationship to violence. Some researchers (84-88) have found that economic inequality reflected in relative deprivation is related to violence because it stimulates hostility in the person who perceives himself to be disadvantaged relative to others. Other researchers (87-89) have found that economic inequality is not related to violence. Instead, they have found that absolute poverty is related to violence and other criminal behavior.

These contradictory results are probably due to the use of large standard metropolitan statistical areas as units of analysis. Such areas are often heterogeneous; for example, one such area contains both suburban Long Island and central Manhattan. A recent study by Messner and Tardiff (90) used neighborhoods that were more naturalistic as smaller units for analysis to test the hypothesis that economic inequality is related to homicide. The findings indicate that economic inequality and race were not related to homicide. Rather, the prime determinants were two: absolute poverty, defined as the percentage of persons below 75 percent of the poverty line, and marital disruption, defined as the percentage of persons separated or divorced. This raises the possibility of the existence of a vicious cycle involving an inability to secure basic necessities of life; disruption of marriage; the production of a single-parent family; increased unemployment; and further difficulty in maintaining interpersonal ties, family structure, and social control. An obviously weighed factor in this conceptualization is the effect of massive unemployment, which (91) has been found to have a causal relationship with crime.

Yet projects such as those of the Vera Institute of Justice in New York City (92) have shown that providing jobs alone, even if one could do so over an extended period of time for the entire group, does not decrease crime including violence. Rather, the basic social system must be addressed. For example, the Eisenhower Foundation has sought to intervene in a comprehensive way by rehabilitating a block of row homes in the inner city areas of Philadelphia in addition to developing positive family and neighborhood structures and attitudes (including Black pride) as well as jobs supported by the local business community. Attempts to evaluate these programs indicate that they are successful, but these have not been systematic, controlled research studies (93).

SUMMARY

The primary prevention of homicide cannot rest on knowledge of discrete biological causes because such knowledge does not exist. Obviously, continued research into biological factors is essential. However, for now the prevention of homicide must be rooted in clinical practice and in socioeconomic changes in society. Psychiatric patients represent only a small proportion of perpetrators of homicide. But attention must be paid to those with a history of violence to determine ways of predicting future violence and homicide and preventing it. Strategies could include mandatory aftercare and protection of potential victims. Another worthwhile approach is to intervene with victims of child abuse to prevent them from becoming violent adults. Prevention programs should also be aimed at parents who are at high risk of abusing their children. These include the single parent, the teenage parent, parents lacking social and economic support, and parents having a child who is handicapped or sick. Interventions intended to prevent or decrease alcohol or drug abuse will decrease homicide and other violence associated with alcohol and drug abuse.

Gun control legislation has the potential to decrease homicides, particularly those involving disputes between family and friends. However, it is doubtful that gun control legislation will decrease homicides related to drug dealing and other criminal activities. Keeping persons with histories of significant violence in prisons for longer periods of time will obviously decrease the rate of homicide, at least in society. However, the legal and ethical dilemmas posed by such selective incarceration are numerous and not readily addressed in this chapter. There is some evidence that early arrests of spouse abusers may decrease subsequent abuse; further research in this area is necessary before we adopt a law and order approach rather than a psychotherapeutic approach to spouse abuse.

Further research is also indicated on the effect of the mass media on violence and homicide rates. This research should be in naturalistic settings and should focus on the long-term effect of the mass media on violent behavior. However, common sense dictates that we not wait for the verdict to be in before lobbying for decreased gratuitous violence on television and in the motion pictures. Finally, efforts must be made to interrupt the cycle of poverty, unemployment, and dissolution of family and social structures particularly prevalent in Black populations in metropolitan areas. Some of these interventions fall within our area of expertise as mental health professionals, but all lie within our responsibility as citizens.

REFERENCES

1. Farley R: Homicide trends in the United States. Demography 17:177-188, 1980
2. Holinger PC: Violent deaths as a leading cause of mortality: an

epidemiological study of suicide, homicide, and accidents. Am J Psychiatry 137:472-476, 1980
3. Klebba J: Homicide trends in the United States, 1900-74. Public Health Rep 90:195-204, 1975
4. Weiss N: Recent trends in violent deaths among young adults in the United States. Am J Epidemiol 103:416-422, 1976
5. Akiyama Y: Murder victimization: a statistical analysis. FBI Law Enforcement Bulletin 50:8-11, 1981
6. Bullock HA: Urban homicide in theory and fact. Journal of Criminal Law, Criminology, and Police Science 45:565-575, 1955
7. Pokorny AD: A comparison of homicide in two cities. Journal of Criminal Law, Criminology, and Police Science 56:479-487, 1965
8. Wolfgang ME: Patterns of Criminal Homicide. New York, Wiley, 1958
9. Voss HL, Hepburn JR: Patterns in criminal homicide in Chicago. Journal of Criminal Law, Criminology, and Police Science 59:499-508, 1968
10. Block B, Zimring RE: Homicide in Chicago. Journal of Research in Crime and Delinquency 10:1-12, 1973
11. Herjanic M, Meyers DA: Notes on epidemiology of homicide in an urban area. Forensic Science 8:235-245, 1976
12. Rushforth NB, Ford AM, Hirsch LS, et al: Violent death in a metropolitan county. N Engl J Med 297:531-538, 1977
13. Constantino JP, Kuller LH, Perper JA, et al: An epidemiological study of homicides in Allegheny County, Pennsylvania. Am J Epidemiol 106:314-324, 1977
14. Tardiff K, Gross E, Messner S: A study of homicide in Manhattan, 1981. Am J Public Health 76:139-143, 1986
15. Hill D, Watterson D: Electroencephalographic studies of psychopathic personalities. J Neurol Neurosurg Psychiatry 5:47-65, 1942
16. Williams D: Neural factors related to habitual aggression. Brain 92:503-520, 1969
17. Sayed ZA, Lewis SA, Brittain RP: An electroencephalographic and psychiatric study of thirty-two insane murderers. Br J Psychiatry 115:1115-1124, 1969
18. Mark VH, Ervin FR: Violence and the Brain. New York, Harper and Row, 1970
19. Hermann BP, Whitman S: Behavioral and personality correlates of epilepsy: a review, methodological critique, and conceptual model. Psychol Bull 95:451-497, 1984
20. Lewis DO, Shanok SS, Pincus JH, et al: Violent juvenile delinquents: psychiatric, neurological, psychological, and abuse

factors. J Am Acad Child Psychiatry 18:307-319, 1979
21. Mednick SA, Volavka J: Biology and crime, in Crime and Justice: An Annual Review of Research (Volume 2). Edited by Morris N, Touny M. Chicago, University of Chicago Press, 1980
22. Bohman M: Some genetic aspects of alcoholism and criminality. Arch Gen Psychiatry 35:269-276, 1978
23. Hutchings B, Mednick SA: Criminality in adoptees and their biological parents: a pilot study, in Biosocial Bases of Criminal Behavior. Edited by Mednick SA, Christiansen KO. New York, Gardner, 1977
24. Schiavi RC, Theilgaard A, Owen DR, et al: Sex chromosome abnormalities hormones, and aggressivity. Arch Gen Psychiatry 41:93-99, 1984
25. Ehrenkranz J, Bliss E, Sheard MH: Plasma testosterone: correlation with aggressive behavior and social dominance in man. Psychosom Med 36:469-475, 1974
26. Kreuz IE, Rose RM: Assessment of aggressive behavior and plasma testosterone in a young criminal population. Psychosom Med 34:321-332, 1972
27. Matthews R: Testosterone levels in aggressive offenders, in Psychopharmacology of Aggression. Edited by Sandler M. New York, Raven, 1979
28. Mattsson A, Schalling D, Olwens D, et al: Plasma 21 testosterone, aggressive behavior, and personality dimensions in young male delinquents. J Am Acad Child Psychiatry 19:476-490, 1980
29. d'Orban PT, Dalton J: Violent crime and the menstrual cycle. Psychol Med 10:353-359, 1980
30. Reid RL, Yen SC: Premenstrual syndrome. Am J Obstet Gynecol 139:85-104, 1981
31. Brown GL, Goodwin FK, Ballenger JC, et al: Aggression in humans: correlates with cerebrospinal fluid amine metabolites. Psychiatry Res 1:131-139, 1979
32. Brown GL, Ebert MH, Goyer PF, et al: Aggression, suicide and serotonin: relationship to CSF amine metabolites. Am J Psychiatry 136:741-746, 1982
33. Lidberg L, Tuck JR, Asberg M, et al: Homicide, suicide and CSF 5-HIAA. Acta Psychiatr Scand 71:230-236, 1985
34. Linnoila M, Virkkunen M, Scheinin M, et al: Low cerebrospinal fluid 5-hydroxyindoleacetic acid concentration differentiates impulsive from nonimpulsive violent behavior. Life Sciences 33:2609-2614, 1983
35. Tardiff K, Sweillam A: Assault, suicide and mental illness. Arch Gen Psychiatry 37:164-169, 1980

36. Tardiff K, Sweillam A: Assaultive behavior among chronic inpatients. Am J Psychiatry 139:212-215, 1982
37. Tardiff K: Characteristics of assaultive patients in private psychiatric hospitals. Am J Psychiatry 22 141:1232-1235, 1984
38. Tardiff K, Koenigsberg HW: Assaultive behavior among psychiatric outpatients. Am J Psychiatry 142:960-963, 1985
39. Craig TJ: An epidemiological study of problems associated with violence among psychiatric inpatients. Am J Psychiatry 139:1262-1266, 1982
40. Yesavage JA, Werner PD, Becker J, et al: Inpatient evaluation of aggression in psychiatric patients. J Nerv Ment Dis 196:299-302, 1981
41. Lion JR, Reid WH (Editors): Assault Within Psychiatric Facilities. New York, Grune and Stratton, 1984
42. McDonald A, Paitrich D: A study of homicide: the validity of predictive test factors. Can J Psychiatry 26:549-554, 1981
43. Langevin R, Paitrich D, Orchard L, et al: Diagnosis of killers seen for psychiatric assessment: a controlled study. Acta Psychiatr Scand 66:216-228, 1982
44. Beck JC (Editor): The Potentially Violent Patient and the Tarasoff Decision in Psychiatric Practice. Washington, DC, American Psychiatric Press, 1985
45. Straus MA, Gelles RJ, Steinmetz SK: Behind Closed Doors: Violence in the American Family. New York, Doubleday/Anchor, 1980
46. Steinmetz SK: The Cycle of Violence: Assertive, Aggressive, and Abusive Family Interaction. New York, Praeger, 1977
47. Kempe CH, Helfer R (Editors): The Battered Child Syndrome (Third Edition). Chicago, University of Chicago Press, 1980
48. Friedrich WN, Boriskin BA: The role of the child in abuse: a review of the literature. Am J Orthopsychiatry 46:580-589, 1976
49. Garbardino J, Sherman D: High-risk neighborhoods and high-risk families: the human ecology of child maltreatment. Child Dev 51:188-198, 1980
50. Daniel JH, Hampton RL, Newberger EH, et al: Child abuse and accidents in black families: a controlled comparative study. Am J Orthopsychiatry 53:645-653, 1983
51. Gladston R: Preventing the abuse of little children: the parents' center project for the study and prevention of child abuse. Am J Orthopsychiatry 45:372-381, 1975
52. Olivens D: Stability of aggressive reaction patterns in males: a review. Psychol Bull 56:313-317, 1963
53. Goodwin J: Family violence: principles of intervention and prevention. Hosp Community Psychiatry 36:1074-1079, 1985

54. Tinklenberg JR: Alcohol and violence, in Alcoholism: Progress in Research and Treatment. Edited by Bourne P, Fox R. New York, Academic Press, 1973
55. Pernanen K: Alcohol and crimes of violence, in The Biology of Alcoholism. Edited by Kissin B, Begleiter H. New York, Plenum, 1976
56. Mayer KE: The Psychobiology of Aggression. New York, Harper and Row, 1976
57. Mendelson JH, Mello NK: Biological concomitants of alcoholism. N Engl J Med 301:912-921, 1979
58. Ellinwood EHl: Assault and homicide associated with amphetamine abuse. Am J Psychiatry 127:1170-1175, 1971
59. Fauman MA, Fauman BJ: Violence associated with phencyclidine abuse. Am J Psychiatry 136:1584=1586, 1979
60. Tinklenberg JR, Murphy PL, Murphy P, et al: Drug involvement in criminal assaults by adolescents. Arch Gen Psychiatry 30:685-689, 1974
61. Wetli CU: Changing patterns of methaqualone abuse: a survey of 246 fatalities. JAMA 249:621-626, 1983
62. Monforte JR, Spitz WU: Narcotic abuse among homicide victims in Detroit. J Forensic Sci 5:186-190, 1974
63. Haberman, PW, Baden MM: Alcohol, Other Drugs, and Violent Death. New York, Oxford University Press, 1978
64. Jason J, Strauss LT, Tyler CW: A comparison of primary and secondary homicides in the United States. Am J Epidemiol 117:309-319, 1983
65. Cook PJ: The role of firearms in violent crime: an interpretive review of the literature, in Criminal Violence. Edited by Wolfgang ME, Weiner NA. Beverly Hills, CA, Sage, 1982
66. Newton GD, Zimring FE: Firearms and Violence in American Life. Washington, DC, U.S. Government Printing Office, 1969
67. Fisher J: Homicide in Chicago: the role of firearms. Criminology 14:387-400, 1976
68. Block R: Violent Crime. Lexington, MA, DC Heath, 1977
69. Zimring F: Firearms and federal law: the Gun Control Act of 1968. Journal of Legal Studies 4:133-198, 1975
70. Deutsch SJ: Intervention modeling: analysis of changes in crime rates. Frontiers in Quantitative Criminology. New York, Academic Press, 1980
71. Jones ED: The District of Columbia's Firearms Control Regulations Act of 1975: the toughest handgun control law in the United States-or is it? Annals of the American Academy of Political and Social Science 5:135-139, 1981
72. Ehrlich I: The deterrent effect of capital punishment: a question of life and death. American Economics Review 65:397-

417, 1975
73. Blumstein A, Cohen J, Nagin D (Editors): Deterrence and Incapacitation: Estimating the Effects of Criminal Sanctions on Crime Rates. Washington, DC, National Academy of Sciences, 1978
74. Kleck G: Capital punishment, gun ownership and homicide. Am J Sociology 84:882-910, 1979
75. Moore MH, Estrich SR, McGillis D, et al: Dangerous Offenders: The Elusive Target of Justice. Cambridge, MA, Harvard University Press, 1984
76. Sherman CW, Berk RA: The specific deterrent effects of arrest for domestic assaults. American Sociological Review 49:261-272, 1984
77. Felthous AR: Crisis intervention in interpartner abuse. Bull Am Acad Psychiatry Law 11:249-260, 1983
78. National Institute of Mental Health: Television and Behavior: 10 Years of Scientific Progress and Implications for the Eighties. Washington, DC, U.S. Government Printing Office, 1982
79. Freedman JL: Effect of television violence on aggressiveness. Psychol Bull 96:227-246, 1984
80. Shotland RL, Goodstein LI: The role of bystanders in crime control. Journal of Social Issues 40:9-26, 1984
81. Messner S, Tardiff K: The social ecology of urban homicide: an application of the "routine activities" approach. Criminology 23:241-267, 1985
82. Silberman CE: Criminal Violence, Criminal Justice. New York, Vintage, 1980
83. Centerwall BS: Race, socioeconomic status and domestic homicide: Atlanta, 1971-72. Am J Public Health 74:813-815, 1984
84. Vold GV: Theoretical Criminology. New York, Oxford University Press, 1979
85. Loftin C, Hill H: Regional subcultures and homicide: an examination of the Gastil-Hackney thesis. American Sociological Review 39:714-724, 1974
86. Blau JR, Blau PM: The cost of inequality: metropolitan structure and violent crime. American Sociological Review 47:114-129, 1982
87. Ehrlich I: Participation in illegitimate activities: a theoretical and empirical investigation. Journal of Political Economy 81:521-565, 1973
88. DeFronzo J: Economic assistance to impoverished Americans: relationship to incidence of crime. Criminology 21:119-136, 1983

89. Williams K: Economic sources of homicide: reestimating the effects of poverty and inequality. American Sociological Review 49:283-289, 1984

90. Messner S, Tardiff K: Economic inequality and levels of homicide: an analysis of urban neighborhoods. Criminology, in press

91. Thornberry TP, Christenson RC: Unemployment and criminal involvement: an investigation of reciprocal causal structures. American Sociological Review 49:398-411, 1984

92. Sviridoff M, McElroy JE: Unemployment and Crime: A Summary Report. New York, Vera Institute of Justice, 1985

93. Curtis L: American Violence and Public Policy. New Haven, CT, Yale University Press, 1985

8

A Discussion of the Prevention of
Alcohol and Drug Abuse and Mental Disorders

Donald I. Macdonald, M.D.

8

A Discussion of the Prevention of Alcohol and Drug Abuse and Mental Disorders

The many issues related to primary prevention raised in the preceding chapters of this monograph are thought provoking and reflect the substantial growth of prevention activities being directed at alcohol and drug abuse and mental disorders (ADM) at all levels of our society. I offer my perspective as both a pediatrician who was until recently in private practice and the head of the Federal program devoted to reducing and preventing alcohol and drug abuse and mental disorders.

Over the last decade, there has been increasing concern within the Federal government, Congress, and the nation regarding the heavy human toll and economic losses associated with ADM disorders. These problems have been estimated to cost the nation $190 billion annually (1). Mental disorders afflict one in every five persons in the United States within a six-month period (2). The abuse of alcohol and drugs, particularly by our nation's youth, has been recognized as a national problem of epidemic proportions. Personal and social costs of alcohol and drug abuse resemble those of major physical illnesses, such as cardiovascular disease and cancer (1).

Since the turn of the century, mortality rates in the general population have steadily declined, and life expectancy has increased. However, for one age group, 15- to 24-year-olds, mortality rates have increased significantly since the early 1960s. Traffic accidents, other accidental trauma, suicide, and homicide constitute the major health threat to adolescents and young adults, accounting for approximately three-quarters of all mortality in this population (3). All of these leading causes of death and disability among young people are preventable. The contribution of alcohol and drug abuse to traffic deaths, to suicide and homicide, and to other tragedies among young Americans cannot be denied.

PREVENTING ALCOHOL AND DRUG
ABUSE AND MENTAL DISORDERS

Conviction has grown among psychiatrists, other ADM professionals, parent groups, government agencies at all levels, and many others that real success can be achieved in reducing the mortality, morbidity, and economic costs associated with ADM disorders if we systematically apply demonstrably effective and affordable prevention programs before the onset of these disorders. In response to this conviction, the Alcohol, Drug Abuse, and Mental Health Administration (ADAMHA) has begun to address the numerous conceptual, methodological, programmatic, and policy issues related to developing, implementing, evaluating, and disseminating viable strategies for reducing the incidence and prevalence of ADM disorders in the population (4, 5).

Drs. Bloom, Puig-Antich, and Goldstein and Asarnow, in Chapters 1, 4, and 5 of this monograph, respectively, outline succinctly some of the conceptual and methodological issues critical to achieving the goals of preventing ADM disorders.

A Decade of Efforts

Since the mid-1970s, ADAMHA has been systematically examining all available public health models of disease prevention and health promotion for their applicability to reducing the incidence and prevalence of ADM disorders. The agency has done so in a carefully considered and deliberate fashion because of the need to weigh the similarities and dissimilarities between ADM disorders and the physical disorders that have been most responsive to prevention strategies, for example, poliomyelitis, smallpox, and measles. Prevention efforts have been most successful in cases in which a specific cause of a disease has been identified, its course understood, and interruption of one or both of these factors accomplished in a cost-effective, efficient manner with minimal negative side-effects.

Not unlike many of the physical diseases, the ADM disorders are characterized by physiological, behavioral, and social aspects. The etiologies of the ADM disorders may, however, be somewhat more complex than those of many physical disorders, and their course of development from onset to manifest disorder may occur over longer spans of time, necessitating a longitudinal framework analogous to the studies summarized by Drs. Goldstein and Asarnow in Chapter 5.

This monograph confirms the general applicability of the traditional public health model of prevention to the ADM disorders and presents numerous examples (see Chapter 5) of prevention approaches that are tailored to specific populations, in specific settings and during specific developmental stages or phases (4).

As an important component of the nation's overall prevention action, the U.S. Public Health Service in 1977 undertook an intensive planning effort focused on three major elements of health promotion and disease prevention--lifestyle, environment, and personal preventive health services. A comprehensive report entitled "Healthy People: The Surgeon General's Report on Health Promotion and Disease Prevention" (3) emerged from this effort. This report emphasizes that major improvements in the health status of Americans can occur through individual health-related behavioral changes and changes in the environment.

This landmark report also expresses an emerging consensus among scientists and health professionals:

There are three overwhelming reasons why a new strong emphasis on prevention--at all levels of government and by all our citizens--is essential . . . prevention saves lives . . . prevention improves the quality of life . . . [and prevention] can save dollars in the long-run. (3, p. 9)

1990 Objectives

In the fall of 1980, the Department of Health and Human Services published a companion document to "Healthy People." The new report, "Promoting Health/Preventing Disease: Objectives for the Nation" (9), provides specific and measurable objectives in 15 priority areas for improving the nation's health by 1990. Of the 15 priority areas, two fall mainly under the mandate of the ADAMHA. The National Institute of Mental Health has the lead institute responsibility for the objective "control of stress and violent behavior."

We do not yet know the specific etiology of many of the ADM disorders, but we do know that stress plays a mediating role in their pathogenesis. Prevention efforts need to be directed toward the control of stress in our daily lives so that we can function better as parents, workers, friends, and neighbors. In Chapter 7 of this monograph, Dr. Tardiff outlines the need for specific intervention to prevent violence and homicide in specific environmental settings and reminds us of the need for careful detection of at-risk populations. Social support, sense of community, and self-help opportunities are emphasized frequently throughout this monograph as important ingredients in any preventive intervention strategy.

The National Institute of Alcohol Abuse and Alcoholism and the National Institute on Drug Abuse have the lead responsibility for the 1990 objective "alcohol and drug misuse prevention." It is encouraging to note that the nation had already met or was well on its way to achieving several of the alcohol/drug abuse goals by 1985. These goals include:

● The proportion of adolescents 12 to 17 years old who abstain from using alcohol or other drugs should not fall below the 1977 level.
● The proportion of young adolescents 18 to 25 years old reporting frequent use of drugs (other than alcohol or tobacco) should not exceed 1977 levels.
● The proportion of adolescents 12 to 17 years old reporting frequent use of drugs (other than alcohol or tobacco) should not exceed 1977 levels.

Data from the National Survey on Drug Abuse (10) and the National Institute on Drug Abuse annual surveys of drug use by high school seniors (11) indicate that these objectives have been met with respect to marijuana and that real progress is being made on other drugs such as sedatives, tranquilizers, and even heroin. Continuing and steadfast prevention efforts are required to maintain this progress, as well as to make similar inroads against persisting problems such as use of cocaine and the newly available and highly dangerous "designer drugs."

The ADAMHA also is involved in meeting the Department of Health and Human Services's objectives "improved nutrition" and "physical fitness and exercise." Dr. Bloom, in Chapter 1 of this monograph, appropriately sees improving nutrition, encouraging physical exercise, and decreasing dependence on alcohol and drugs as targets ripe for further prevention activities. Drs. Frances and Franklin, in Chapter 6, suggest an impressive number of settings where primary prevention activities addressing these disorders can be implemented. Among the approaches are school-based educational programs, mass media techniques (TV and radio), and workplace programs. Their notion of early identification and intervention with high risk populations is one that is being pursued by ADAMHA as it supports the development of interventions for children of emotionally disturbed parents, children of alcoholics, children with chronic physical illnesses, the elderly, and minority populations (12, 13). Drs. Munoz, Chan, and Armus provide a well-reasoned discussion of the need to be particularly sensitive to the vulnerabilities of minority populations and populations in transition in Chapter 2.

Role of Life-Style

Many recent studies and reports, most notably the report on research in biobehavioral sciences by the National Academy of Sciences Institute of Medicine (14), have pointed out that many ADM disorders can be seen as the result of personal adjustments to stressful life events, occupational demands, and life-style changes. As discussed by Dr. Eisenberg in Chapter 3 of this monograph, Drs. Goldstein and Asarnow in Chapter 5, and Dr. Bloom in Chapter 1, prevention interventions can be developed and implemented to address these variables and consequences and include the role of social support networks and community involvement. In 1979, the Centers for Disease Control analyzed the 10 leading causes of death in the United States in regard to their contributing factors. They concluded that 50 percent of the proportional allocation of the contributing factors to mortality was due to life-style issues. An additional 25 percent of the contributing factors were related to environmental conditions (15).

Of pressing concern, as noted by Drs. Bloom, Eisenberg, and Puig-Antich (Chapters 1, 3, and 4, respectively) is the need to address self-destructive life-styles. For example, increases in adolescent and young adult suicide rates in the United States illustrate the need to move forward in developing effective prevention programs. The National Institute of Mental Health has established a suicide prevention program that is actively working with state, community, and parent groups to develop effective approaches for reducing this tragic loss of life. Similarly, ADAMHA has undertaken an initiative to further educate primary care givers about ADM disorders in order to improve their abilities in early detection, identification, and treatment of these disorders. The education of the public, especially concerned parent groups, about vulnerability to ADM disorders is a high priority for us and truly within the public health model of primary prevention. References are made to activities, conferences, and research projects supported by the ADAMHA institutes in Chapters 1, 5, 6, and 7.

Recent Accomplishments

A review of some recent ADAMHA prevention accomplishments is pertinent to this discussion.

For the first time, the agency has established the position of Associate Administrator for Prevention, the responsibilities of which include coordinating agency-wide prevention activities and advising the ADAMHA Administrator on current and future developments related to prevention of ADM disorders.

The Second Annual Prevention Activities Report is a comprehensive outline of all prevention activities of the ADAMHA. The first report showed that in Fiscal Year 1983, the agency invested more than $14.7 million in prevention activities. In Fiscal Year 1984, the figure was $21 million. This was approximately 10 percent of the overall research budget, and represented an increase of 42 percent over 1983.

The ADAMHA convened a prevention roundtable of outside experts in October 1984 to recommend an agenda of needed prevention activities in the alcohol and drug abuse areas for the coming months and years. Among the activities recommended was a convening of a national conference on prevention of alcohol and drug problems, scheduled for August 1986, with the aim of expediting application of new prevention research findings. The National Institute on Alcohol Abuse and Alcoholism and the National Institute on Drug Abuse will develop regional prevention workshops to follow up the national conference with further technical assistance for implementing innovative prevention approaches. In addition, the two institutes will convene joint and separate expert consensus panels to review the state of the art in selected prevention areas and suggest further directions for research.

In another development, Congress passed legislation (the Alcohol, Drug Abuse, and Mental Health Amendments of 1984) that established a 15-member Alcohol, Drug Abuse, and Mental Health Advisory Board, with a requirement that a minimum of six members have expertise in ADM prevention and education. This advisory group is providing valuable input for the agency's prevention work.

CONCLUSION

The importance of strong prevention efforts, especially in early and mid-adolescence, cannot be overstressed. Substance use patterns are begun at this time of life and have a pervasive influence on subsequent behaviors. Primary prevention aimed at these youngsters can go a long way toward mitigating or eliminating these problems in further generations. Kandel has shown in long-term studies (16) that once drug use has begun, there is a clear pattern of progression from "gateway" drugs such as alcohol, tobacco, and marijuana to other illicit drugs and to abuse of prescription psychoactive drugs in young adulthood. It is well documented that alcohol and drug abuse are etiologic or precipitating factors in many medical as well as psychiatric illnesses. Substance abuse was found to be a major factor in 40 percent of inpatient admissions and 50 percent of emergency room visits in two teaching hospitals (17). Psychiatrists, pediatricians, primary practitioners, and all health workers should reappraise their practices in light of what is happening to today's youth and take action to identify and intervene to prevent ADM problems at the earliest possible moment.

REFERENCES

1. Harwood HJ, Napolitano DM, Kristiansen PL, et al: Economic Costs to Society of Alcohol and Drug Abuse and Mental Illness: 1980 (Contract No. ADM 283-83-0002). Research Triangle Park, NC, Research Triangle Institute, 1984
2. Regier DA, Myers JK, Kramer M, et al: The NIMH Epidemiological Catchment Area Program. Arch Gen Psychiatry 41: 934-941, 1984
3. U.S. Department of Health, Education, and Welfare: Healthy People: The Surgeon General's Report on Health Promotion and Disease Prevention (DHEW Publication No. 79-55071). Washington, DC, U.S. Government Printing Office, 1979
4. Alcohol, Drug Abuse, and Mental Health Administration: Report to Congress of the Prevention Activities of the Alcohol, Drug Abuse and Mental Health Administration, Fiscal Year 1983. Washington, DC, U.S. Government Printing Office, 1984
5. Alcohol, Drug Abuse, and Mental Health Administration. ADAMHA Prevention Policy and Programs 1979-1982 (DHHS Publication No. ADM 81-1038). Washington, DC, U.S. Government Printing Office, 1981
6. Klein DC, Goldston SE (Editors): Primary Prevention: An Idea Whose Time Has Come (DHHS Publication No. ADM 77-447). Washington, DC, U.S. Government Printing Office, 1977
7. Engel GL: The need for a new medical model: a challenge for biomedicine. Science 196:129-136, 1977
8. National Institute of Mental Health: Center for Prevention Research Annual Report. Rockville, MD, National Institute of Mental Health, 1983
9. U.S. Department of Health and Human Services. Promoting Health/Preventing Disease: Objectives for the Nation. Washington, DC, U.S. Government Printing Office, 1980

10. Miller JD, Cisin IH, Gardner-Keaton H, et al: National Survey on Drug Abuse: Main Findings 1982 (DHHS Publication No. ADM 83-1263). Washington, DC, U.S. Government Printing Office, 1983
11. Johnston LD, O'Malley PM, Bachman JA: Use of Licit and Illicit Drugs by America's High School Students: 1975-1984 (DHHS Publication No. ADM 84-1394).Washington, DC, U.S. Government Printing Office, 1985
12. Silverman MM: Preventive intervention research: a new beginning, in Southeast Asian Mental Health: Treatment, Prevention, Services, Training, and Research (DHHS Publication No. ADM 85-1399). Edited by Owan T. Washington, DC, U.S. Government Printing Office, 1985
13. Silverman MM, Levin VS: Research on the prevention of psychological disorders of infancy: a federal perspective, in New Directions in Failure to Thrive: Implications for Research and Practice. Edited by Drotar D. New York, Plenum Press, 1985
14. Hamburg D, Elliott GR, Parron DL: Health and Behavior: Frontiers of Research in the Biobehavioral Sciences. Washington, DC, National Academy Press, 1982
15. Centers for Disease Control. Ten Leading Causes of Death, 1977. Atlanta, GA, 1980
16. Kandel DB, Logan, JA: Patterns of drug use from adolescence to young adulthood. Periods of risk for initiation, continued use, and discontinuation. Am J Public Health 74:660-666, 1984
17. Kamerow DB, Pincus HA, Macdonald DI: Alcohol abuse, other drug abuse, and mental disorders in medical practice: prevalence, costs, recognition, and treatment. JAMA 225:2054-2057, 1986

9

Issues to Consider in
Primary Prevention in Psychiatry

Steven S. Sharfstein, M.D.

9

Issues to Consider in
Primary Prevention in Psychiatry

Primary prevention as a concept and as a field of inquiry has matured considerably since my days 15 years ago as a director of a mental health program in a neighborhood health center. Part of the justification for establishing a neighborhood health program with a comprehensive mental health service were the concepts of primary and secondary prevention. By being close to the lives of patients and families, one might be able to develop prevention programs for individuals at risk and effectively intervene early enough in the cycle of illness and disability to prevent long-term and more severe illness.

I recall two experiences that created some skepticism on my part about prevention. The first was clearly related to the news in the community of my arrival as a full-time psychiatrist in a health program. At that point the human service people, for example the welfare worker and the school truant officer, immediately began to send their troubled clients to me for evaluation and possible treatment. The number of clients sent was staggering. Eventually I was receiving two or three referrals a day from the truant officer even as I was interacting with the primary care providers and caseworkers in this working-class community around a range of mental health and general health problems of a large caseload. I immediately learned that the best strategy was to call up the truant officer and the welfare worker who seemed to be indiscriminately referring clients to me and ask for a regular time to meet with them in order to discuss their caseload and most troubled clients. This was part of my consultation role in the community, but I saw it as a prevention program, in the sense that it prevented my being overwhelmed by cases that I could not possibly diagnose or treat!

The second experience concerned an activist pediatrician who received a grant from the Commonwealth of Massachusetts to screen the 900 school children in our neighborhood for a range of physical and mental disabilities. He was able to hire nurses to go into the schools, work with the teachers, and do a comprehensive evaluation. Again, my concern was that we would be identifying many children for whom we could not possibly provide services. Despite my concerns about this, and the raised expectations of many parents in the community, the team of screeners came to me to report that of the 900 children who had been tested, 600 required mental diagnosis and treatment. The pediatrician chimed in that they were able to assess the severity of the problems and had identified the 50 most severe who required some immediate attention. At that point, I indicated that we were able to assess approximately one a week. This of course created a fair amount of consternation in the community, which warned me about the possible adverse impact of early screening and evaluation.

Despite these experiences on the front lines, I have retained an abiding belief in the cost effectiveness of preventive activity and its distinct human value. The chapters in this monograph underscore the promise as well as some of the major accomplishments in the field of prevention and their potential application in programs such as the one that I described--a combination of primary health care and mental health care in a community at high risk.

I believe strongly, in agreement with Dr. Bloom (see Chapter 1 of this monograph), that the shift from disease-specific models to integrated delivery system and biopsychosocial models is a salutatory one. The interdependency of physical and mental disorders is now clearly established, and there is an accumulation of research on cost offsets due to decreased use of medical care with the provision of mental health care (1). This has an immediate impact on questions of payment, especially in this era of prospective payment and diagnosis-related groups. Consultation/liaison psychiatry, for example, promises a cost-effective clinical intervention that will lead to shorter lengths of stay and a lower use of medical services in the hospital for patients who have only a fixed amount available to pay for their episode of care. Life event stress theory, the concept of generic illness, and the importance of social supports all support this particularly effective conceptualization.

The nonspecific intervention issue receives further credence by Dr. Eisenberg in Chapter 3 of this monograph. Economic progress that improves the diet as well as the quality of water and other factors also improves the mental health of the public. An interesting concern, however, when one considers some of the prevention issues in the over-65 age group. When the goal is merely to lengthen life and not increase productivity, the cost benefit of the intervention comes under question. For some age groups the most cost-effective medical intervention would be to either cure the illness or let the patient die and not have a prolonged course of costly suffering. Most of medical care, however, takes the form of "halfway technologies," to paraphrase Dr. Louis Thomas (2), which costs more in both the short and long run. Much of our investment in intensive care units in general hospitals and high-cost diagnostic and intervention technologies such as computer axial tomography and coronary bypass surgery come under this rubric. So, too, for psychiatric care, particularly as it relates to those over age 65. Yet the cost-benefit issues only emphasize the need to take a broader look at the equity of our overall system of health care and provide opportunities for health and life even in the face of dubious potential from a cost-benefit perspective.

Among the most promising areas for nonspecific preventive interventions are family planning and the related areas of safe sex, preschool interventions, and a variety of approaches toward studying the origins of developmental and neurologic problems. The potential preventive impact of gun control on both the suicide and the homicide rate is presented by Dr. Tardiff in Chapter 7 as having significant promise.

Drs. Frances and Franklin report in Chapter 6 on the progress of prevention efforts in the alcohol field. They see potential for preventive interventions in corporate employee assistance programs; with the media, in redirection of beer and other alcoholic beverage commercials; and in increasing the age of legal drinking. Perhaps no other area is more integrative concerning the medical and social consequences of certain actions than the study of alcoholism. A fascinating opportunity for future research lies in the potential to discover biological markers that identify individuals at high risk for alcohol problems and possibly a vaccine against alcoholism and other substance abuse problems.

Close examination of the potential for prevention of serious mental disorders, for example, schizophrenia or affective disorder, reveals that we have a long way to go, despite our considerable progress. The need for investment in basic research on the brain and on the interaction between the environment and the nervous system is clearly evident. We need to know how to put together sophisticated findings in neurointegration with markers of vulnerability in the neurologic and behavioral continuum.

Fifteen years ago, in the middle of my experience at the neighborhood health center, I felt we were floundering in attempts at preventive interventions in mental health. Today I have high hopes and expectations for the future, despite the daunting task of trying to discover the basic mechanisms of mental health and illness or the interaction between the neuron and the environment. In this era of medical care crises precipitated by mindless cost consciousness and cost effectiveness, our investment in research in prevention will pay off many times over.

REFERENCES

1. Mumford E, Schlesinger HJ, Glass GV, et al: A new look at evidence about reduced cost of medical utilization following mental health treatment. Am J Psychiatry 141:1145-1158, 1984
2. Thomas L: Biomedical research and the future of public health. Health Affairs 2:32-40, 1983

PSYCHIATRIC INSTITUTE
LIBRARY

LANGLEY PORTER
PSYCHIATRIC INSTITUTE
LIBRARY